HANDBOOK
OF
INTRAOPERATIVE
MONITORING

Special thanks to Michael D. Maves, M.D.
for serving as Medical Editor and
consultant.

Michael D. Maves, M.D.
Executive Vice-President
American Academy of Otolaryngology—Head
and Neck Surgery
Alexandria, Virginia

HANDBOOK
OF
INTRAOPERATIVE
MONITORING

Edited By

■ DOUGLAS L. BECK, M.A. ■

St. Louis University Health Sciences Center
Department of Otolaryngology—Head and Neck Surgery
St. Louis, Missouri

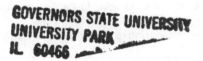

SINGULAR PUBLISHING GROUP, INC.
San Diego, California

Singular Publishing Group, Inc.
4284 41st Street
San Diego, California 92105-1197

© 1994 by Singular Publishing Group, Inc.

Typeset in 10/12 Times Roman by House Graphics
Printed in the United States of America by McNaughton & Gunn

Library of Congress Cataloging-in-Publication Data

Handbook of intraoperative monitoring / edited by Douglas L. Beck.
    p.   cm.
    Includes bibliographical references.
    ISBN 1-56593-210-2
    1. Head—Surgery.   2. Neck—Surgery.   3. Ear—Surgery.
  4. Intraoperative monitoring.   I. Beck, Douglas L.
    [DNLM: 1. Intraoperative Monitoring—handbooks. WO 39 H2354
1994]
    RD521.H36   1994
    617.8——dc20
    DNLM/DLC   94-12881
    for Library of Congress   CIP

■ CONTENTS ■

SECTION TWO: SPINAL CORD MONITORING

SECTION THREE: THE PHYSICIAN'S PERSPECTIVE

■ PREFACE ■

Someone recently asked me, "What was it that got you interested in audiology, was it the money or the fame?" I still chuckle.

It is my hope that this book serves to highlight the role of the audiologist in the operating room. I hope this book allows the audiologist considering this type of work to make a more informed decision, and to have a better idea of expectations and standards as they currently exist. These will certainly change.

With admittedly little preparation, I had the good fortune to be in the right place at the right time. I learned most of what I know about intraoperative monitoring from the physicians and fellows at the Otologic Medical Group and the House Ear Institute in Los Angeles about 10 years ago. I am grateful to them for their knowledge, patience, and patients.

As audiologists we have little or no knowledge about the operating room. Although we are prepared to perform and interpret electrophysiologic tests, applying this knowledge to the operating room is difficult. Although we may have an interest in the operating room, it is difficult to find graduate programs that prepare us to work in this environment (Hall, Schwaber, Henry, & Baer, 1993).

Despite the American Speech-Language-Hearing Association's 1992 scope of practice statement which endorsed audiologists participating in neurophysiologic monitoring, we find ourselves ill-prepared to enter the operating room.

There are turf battles in the operating room—not just among audiologists, nurses, EEG, and E.P. technicians—but between plastic surgeons and facial plastic surgeons, between general surgeons and otolaryngologists, between neurosurgeons and orthopedic surgeons, between anesthetists and anesthesiologists, and on and on. Turf battles are nothing new, and we are not the first professionals engaged in this unpleasant reality. The most distressing part of the battle to me is the observation that audiologists often aim their cannons at other audiologists.

Rather than saying who is not qualified to do what, I'd rather say that, if individuals performing intraoperative monitoring are practicing within their scope of practice as defined by their profession, and if they are appropriately trained (leaving that vague intentionally), they are probably fine. I must admit that this is a flawed way of determining who should perform intraoperative monitoring, but it seems to be the best way possible at this time.

I am opposed to additional licensing for audiologists in the operating room, although I support continuing education and workshop tutorials. I believe that audiologists can be appropriately trained to serve in the operating room by virtue of their graduate studies, the fellowship year, the scope of practice definition issued by the American Speech-Language-Hearing Association, and through the informal mentorship programs that almost everyone participates in.

To me, intraoperative monitoring is like hearing aids, central auditory processing, aural rehabilitation, balance testing, electroneurography, and pediatric testing. The person performing the task must take self-responsibility for maintaining his or her education and abilities. We must limit our practice not only to the limits of our license, but we must practice responsibility within our area of expertise.

I am certainly not capable of working as an expert in all areas of audiology, and I don't know anyone who is. We must pick and choose and actively pursue our areas of expertise just as our colleagues in medicine do.

Unlike the many areas of clinical audiology, the audiologist involved with intraoperative monitoring is never autonomous. The role of the audiologist in the operating room is similar to the scrub nurse, the circulating nurse, the anesthesiologist, the physician's assistant, and other "support personnel" who work in concert to support the efforts of the surgeon in helping the patient.

I am often asked the question, "Is it necessary to have the audiologist do the monitoring? Can't the nurse or the doctor "plug in" the patient and leave the machine on?"

My typical answer includes: Does the surgeon need the scrub nurse? Well, probably not. The surgeon could certainly pick up the instruments and prepare each item.

However, it would slow things down and it would not be efficient. Does the surgeon need the anesthesiologist or the anesthetist? Well, it helps to have someone else knowledgeable about medicine taking care of the patient's vital signs during surgery. But, yes, the surgeon could probably do the anesthesiology job if needed. In fact, the surgeon did a residency rotation through anesthesiology and with rare exception surgeons hardly ever do a rotation through audiology.

Which brings us back to: Does the surgeon need the audiologist? If the surgeon has been trained in audiology or neurophysiology, the likelihood is that he or she could do the monitoring. However, if the surgeons spend their time in the operating room trouble-shooting equipment, turning dials, placing electrodes, and interpreting ongoing EMG or other evoked potential information, then they are not paying 100 percent attention to the most important task—the surgery, itself.

Intraoperative monitoring as a subspecialty area of audiology requires academic knowledge, experience in neurophysiologic monitoring, an extensive background in electrophysiology (best obtained in graduate school), and appropriate training—preferably through a mentorship program. It is foolhardy (and dangerous) to assume that "just plugging in the patient and turning on the machine" is equivalent to having an appropriately trained expert in the room.

Intraoperative monitoring is intense. It is not for everyone. Mistakes made in the operating room may cause pain and suffering for the patient, and these same mistakes are likely to end up in litigation.

It is important to remember that patients do not come into the operating room so that the anesthesiologist can put them to sleep. Likewise, patients do not come into the operating room to be monitored. They come to the operating room to have surgery. As is true with all intraoperative monitoring, the goal is to define and protect structures that are at risk for damage during surgical procedures—whenever possible.

Even the best intraoperative monitoring is no substitute for excellent surgical skill and anatomic knowledge. In the ideal setting, intraoperative monitoring is a tool that enhances the surgeon's knowledge. Intraoperating monitoring can in no way guarantee an excellent surgical result. The primary factor in surgical success is the surgeon's knowledge and skill.

Intraoperative monitoring allows the surgeon to know more about the anatomic structures involved in the surgery, based on the physiologic responses made available via monitoring. The best monitoring in the world will not make a poor surgeon into a good surgeon. However, monitoring can help a good surgeon do a better job.

The book is organized in three sections. The first and second sections are the "how to get it done" sections. They are written almost exclusively by audiologists. The first two sections are not intended to be epic in scope. They are intended to be useful in helping the novice get oriented, be prepared, have references on the subject, and provide a working protocol that accomplishes the goals of intraoperative monitoring. The first section addresses Cranial Nerve Monitoring with the second section addressing Spinal Cord Monitoring. The third section consists of four chapters written by prominent physicians describing the most commonly monitored surgical procedures by the surgeons who perform them, as well as a detailed discussion of anesthesia and its relationship to intraoperative monitoring.

I am eternally grateful to my coauthors for their knowledge, orientation to task, and tolerance through the deadlines, editing, and rewriting. Often I am reminded of my English 101 class, in which the definition of writing was etched into my mind, likely forever: "writing is rewriting."

All of the book's attributes are exclusively due to the efforts of my highly talented coauthors and advisers. The oversights, errors, and unresolved thoughts are entirely mine.

Thanks to Sharon Fitzgerald for most things that go right during the day. Thanks to Michael Maves for serving as medical editor and supporting me through the rough spots. Thanks to Joanne Slater for a thousand other things. Thanks to Marie Linvill and Jeff Danhauer for their gentle prodding and wisdom.

And an extra special thanks to the most wonderful girls in the world, Olivia and Hannah, and their mom, (my wife) Barbara, for the love, devotion, patience, and laughter (Oh, I owe it all to you, you make me happy).

DLB

REFERENCES

Hall, J. W., Schwaber, M. K., Henry, M. M., & Baer, J.E. (1993) Intraoperative monitoring of the auditory system for hearing preservation. *Seminars in Hearing, 14,* (2) 143–154.

American Speech-Language-Hearing Association (ASHA). *Asha, 34,* (Suppl. 7), 1992.

■ CONTRIBUTORS ■

Aukse E. Bankaitis, M.A.
Department of Otolaryngology
University of Cincinnati Medical
  Center
Cincinnati, Ohio

Carl J. Bassi, Ph.D.
School of Optometry
University of Missouri-St. Louis
St. Louis, Missouri

Douglas L. Beck, M.A.
St. Louis University Health Sciences
  Center
Department of Otolaryngology—Head
  and Neck Surgery
St. Louis, Missouri

Derald Brackmann, M.D.
House Ear Clinic, Inc.
Los Angeles, California

Richard Bucholz, M.D.
Department of Neurosurgery
St. Louis University School of
  Medicine
St. Louis, Missouri

Ken Henry, Ph.D.
Falls Church, Virginia

Leslie S. Holland, M.D.
Department of Orthopedic Surgery
Washington University
St. Louis, Missouri

Robert W. Keith, Ph.D.
Department of Otolaryngology
University of Cincinnati Medical
  Center
Cincinnati, Ohio

Sandra B. Kinsella, M.D.
Carmel, Indiana

Gary LaBlance, Ph.D.
St. Louis Children's Hospital
St. Louis, Missouri

Anne Padberg, M.S.
Washington University School of
  Medicine
Division of Orthopedic Surgery
St. Louis, Missouri

Eric W. Sargent, M.D.
Department of Otolaryngology
St. Louis University School of
  Medicine
St. Louis, Missouri

Joanne M. Slater, M.S.
St. Louis University Health Sciences
  Center
Department of Otolaryngology—Head
  and Neck Surgery
St. Louis, Missouri

Ian M. Windmill, Ph.D.
Associate Professor
Myers Hall
University of Louisville School of
  Medicine
Louisville, Kentucky

Karen Yaffee, M.D.
St. Louis University Health Sciences
  Center
Department of Otolaryngology—Head
  and Neck Surgery
St. Louis, Missouri

■ SECTION ONE ■

THE CRANIAL NERVES

■ CHAPTER 1 ■

MONITORING THE OPTIC NERVE

■ CARL J. BASSI, Ph.D. ■

Neurosurgical interventions along the visual pathway put visual function at risk. Horwitz and Rizzoli (1982) report that 19–39% of patients undergoing suprasellar meningioma surgery have a decrease in visual function. The reported rates of visual loss were approximately 4–13% for pituitary adenomas and craniopharyngiomas (Fahlbusch, 1981; Horwitz & Rizzoli, 1982). Reliable methods for monitoring the visual system during surgery might prove beneficial in identifying and preserving vital structures during dissection, excision, or lesion destruction. A number of case studies and larger prospective studies have used visual evoked potentials (VEPs) to monitor surgical procedures along the visual pathway. This chapter critically reviews those studies.

It is widely accepted that changes in latency, phase, and amplitude of the VEP can be used in the clinical assessment of visual function. VEP techniques have been utilized in the assessment of the integrity of the visual pathway (for general reviews see Carr & Siegel, 1990; Regan, 1989), in nonresponsive subjects such as infants (Norcia & Tyler, 1985; Wright, Eriksen, Shors, & Ary, 1986), and in patients with dementia (Pollock, Schneifer, Chui, Henderson, Zemansky, & Sloane, 1989). For VEPs to be useful during intraoperative monitoring (IOM) four conditions are ideal:

1. VEPs can be recorded easily and reliably in the operating room.

2. Decrements in the VEPs during surgery correspond with postoperative sensory deficits.
3. Intraoperative augmentation (maintaining the VEP baseline) in VEPs is not associated with postoperative decrements in vision.
4. Intraoperative VEP changes can be used to warn or prevent sensory deficits.

   This chapter includes an overview of the anatomy of the visual pathways, from retina through extrastriate visual cortex; a review of visual electrodiagnostic testing (especially VEP testing); typical recording and stimulation parameters for IOM of VEPs; a review of studies using VEPs during IOM; and future directions in the use of VEPs during IOM.

ANATOMY OF THE PRIMARY VISUAL PATHWAY

The primary visual pathway (Figure 1-1) consists of the receptor organ (the retina), the pathway from the eye to the lateral geniculate nucleus of the thalamus (optic nerve, chiasm, and tract), the lateral geniculate nucleus, the pathway from lateral geniculate nucleus to the visual cortex (optic radiations), and primary visual cortex (Brodmann's area V1). The retina is a multilayered structure that consists of a photoreceptor outer segment layer, the outer nuclear layer composed of the photoreceptor cell nuclei, the inner nuclear layer (containing horizontal, bipolar, and amacrine cells), and the ganglion cell layer. Axons from the ganglion cell layer exit the eye through the optic disk and contribute to forming the optic nerve. After leaving the eye, axonal fibers from the nasal retina of each eye cross at the optic chiasm. The optic tracts are made up of ganglion cell axons from the ipsilateral temporal retinas and contralateral nasal retinas from each eye. The axons of the optic tract synapse in the lateral geniculate nucleus with geniculate cells, the axons of which form the optic radiations that finally synapse in Layer IV of Brodmann's area V1. There are multiple visual areas located in temporal and parietal cortical regions (DeYoe & VanEssen, 1988; Kaas, 1986).

   This schematic of the primary visual pathway does not include the large number of inputs from the optic nerve to areas such as the suprachiasmatic nucleus, superior colliculus, pulvinar, and hypothalamic nuclei (Sadun, 1986; Sadun, Johnson, & Schaechter, 1986; Sadun, Johnson, & Smith, 1986). In addition, the primary visual pathway comprises a number of parallel visual pathways that have different anatomic, physiologic, and functional properties (for reviews see Bassi & Lehmkuhle, 1990; DeYoe & VanEssen, 1988; Kaas, 1986; Regan, 1989).

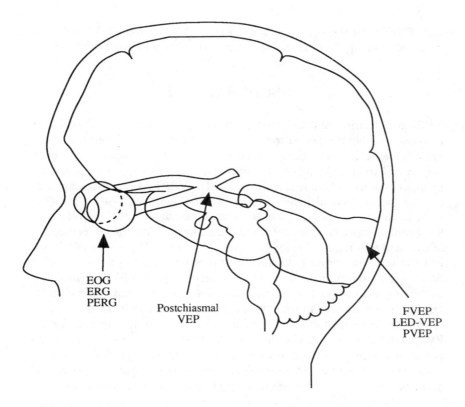

FIGURE 1–1. Schematic of primary visual pathway with electrodiagnostic tests associated with testing different positions.

Figure 1–1 also shows the various electrodiagnostic tests used to assess function along the visual pathway (for a review of tests see Carr & Siegel, 1990). At the retinal level: the electro-oculogram (EOG) is used to assess the retinal pigment epithelium/photoreceptor function, the electroretinogram (ERG) can assess outer retina function (including photoreceptor function with the initial negative A wave component and bipolar and Müller cell function with the later positive component B wave), and the pattern electroretinogram (PERG) can assess ganglion cell function. Postchiasmal function can be assessed with the postchiasmal VEP (Gouras & MacKay, 1988). The posterior visual pathway (including optic nerve, optic tract, optic radiations, and visual cortex) can be assessed with flash (FVEP), LED (LED-VEP), or pattern (PVEP) visual evoked potentials. To date, FVEPs and LED-VEPs have been used principally to assess optic nerve function during surgery.

NONSURGICAL VEPs

VEPs are electrical signals recorded from the occipital cortical region in response to either flash or pattern light stimulation. Unlike the electroretino-gram (a transcleral potential recorded at the cornea) that measures the mass response of voltage changes of the entire retina, the VEP is mainly generated by the central 6 to 12 degrees of the retina. The VEP is of very low amplitude (tens of microvolts) and therefore requires either signal-averaging techniques or other special techniques such as sweep recording to sufficiently improve the signal-to-noise ratio for detection. Flash VEPs (FVEPs) are recorded in response to a light flash. Typically flashes are produced by a xenon flash unit or LED goggles. Typically a ganzfeld stimulus is used to produce an even flash across the entire retina. The advantages of the FVEP/LED-VEP include: (1) the subject does not need to fixate or even attend to the stimulus and (2) there is no need for refractive correction. The disadvantages include: (1) greater between-subject variability in the waveform than that for the PVEP (Halliday, Barret, Caroll, & Kriss, 1982) or other sensory evoked potentials (Grundy, 1982); (2) ganzfeld flash stimulation systems are typical-ly large and interfere with a surgeon's freedom of movement (Wright, Arden, & Jones, 1973); and (3) the flashes can interfere with a surgeon's vision.

Traditional FVEP or LED-VEP interpretations are based on the meas-urement of the amplitudes and latencies of the response components which are often complex sequences of positive and negative voltage peaks. Normal subjects typically have a positive peak at a latency of 60–120 msec for a flash presented to the central retina (Sokol, 1976). The amplitudes of the VEPs are small (typically 3–10 μV); however, the most reliable components of the wave are the first negative peak (N1), the first positive maximum (P1), and the second negative voltage maximum (N2). Typical analyses include measurement of N1, P1, and N2 latencies and the N1/P1 amplitudes. (See Figure 1–2.)

A patterned light stimulus consisting of either alternating checkerboard or sine wave grating stimuli can also be used to elicit VEPs in patients. There is typically less inter- or intrasubject variability in the latency of responses (usually in the 100–120 msec range for high contrast checkerboard stimuli) in most normal patients to patterned stimuli (Halliday et al., 1982). The use of pattern stimuli is often impractical in the operating room with current stimulation systems. The pattern stimuli are difficult to present and focus needs to be maintained under general anesthesia to yield a repeatable VEP. In addition, surgical draping can hinder access to the patient's eyes.

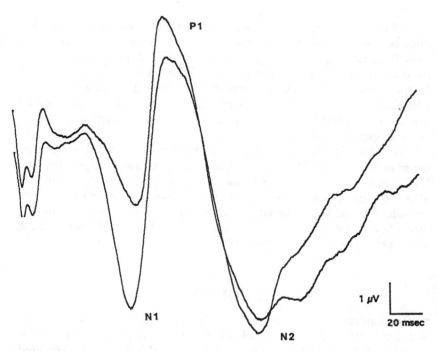

FIGURE 1-2. Example flash visual evoked potential to a ganzfeld flash stimulus presented at 1.4 Hz. Each tracing represents the average of 100 sweeps. The electrode configuration was the same as in Figure 1-3A.

RECOMMENDED STANDARDS FOR IOM OF VEPs (EVOKED POTENTIALS COMMITTEE, 1987)

STIMULATION

The most common stimulus systems are goggles fit with LEDs or modified contact lenses (Harding, Smith, & Yorke, 1987). Both of these sources can provide flash stimuli that can vary in wave length, temporal frequency, and intensity. Care is needed to assure that damage to the eyes does not occur with these stimulation systems. Ocular trauma can occur with either improper goggle placement or movement of the goggles during surgery. Goggles are impractical during anterior cranial fossa surgery because of their size. Risks associated with contact lens stimulators include corneal abrasions and ulcerations. If hard or PMMA lens are used, they should only be used for 30 minutes or less. Risks and contraindications for each stimulus delivery system should be documented by the manufacturer and should be discussed with the patient prior to obtaining surgical consent.

Stimulus intensity calibration can be unreliable, because stimulation is often performed through closed eyelids. However, conditions are kept constant from pre- through postoperative monitoring allowing assessment of interval changes. A stimulus rate of 1–2.5 Hz for single-flash VEPs and 830 Hz for steady-state VEPs is recommended. As retinal illumination can affect stimulus intensity, dilated pupils (by conjunctival mydriatics) should be used to maintain constant retinal illumination. Dilation may be contraindicated for many surgical procedures.

Because of the high intersubject variability of the FVEP, it is necessary to obtain baseline FVEPs before intraoperative recording begins. Because VEPs can be influenced by anesthesia, VEPs should be recorded immediately after the patient is anesthetized. Frequent periodic recording during the procedure should be employed to monitor changes over time. An ongoing dialogue with the anesthesiologist will aid in identification of changes in the VEP to be reported to the surgeon.

RECORDING

System bandpass: A bandpass of 1–300 Hz (–3 dB cutoff) is recommended, with filter rolloff slopes at 12 dB/octave for low frequencies and 24 dB/octave for high frequencies. Digital smoothing and filtering are considered acceptable alternatives.

Analysis time: 250–500 msec.

Averaging: A total of 50–200 trials is recommended. Repeat tracings are necessary to demonstrate the reproducibility of responses.

Electrode type and placement: Typically, standard EEG electrodes are used. These cup electrodes are applied to the scalp with collodion and are sealed with plastic tape. Alternatively, subdermal needle electrodes can be used. These electrodes are quicker to insert, but should not be reused. Impedance should be between 500–5,000 ohm. Typical electrode placements are shown in Figure 1–3. Electrodes are placed over: (1) midline occipital (MO) region, 5 cm above the inion (Oz position of the 10–20 system), (2) over the midline frontal (MF) region 12 cm above the nasion (position Fz of the 10–20 system); and (3) on the earlobes at A1 and A2 (or mastoids). The ground is often placed at the vertex. Often MF and Fz positions are within the surgical field—in which case more posterior midline placements are used.

Montage: A minimum two-channel recording is suggested: channel 1 (active-MO and reference-MF); and channel 2 (active-MO and reference-linked earlobes A1/A2).

Drug effects: Most preanesthetic and anesthetic agents have been shown to change VEP amplitudes (Clark & Rosner, 1973; Domino, 1967).

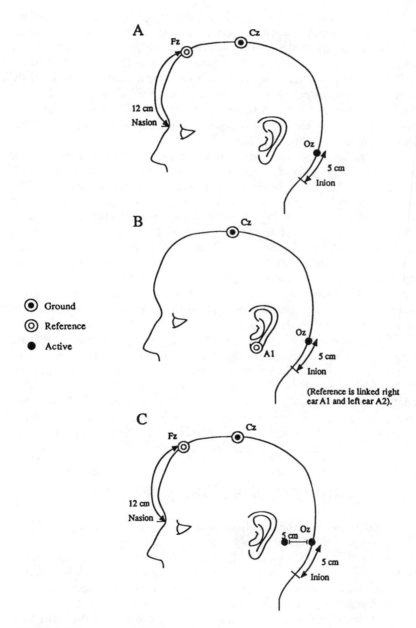

FIGURE 1–3. Example electrode configurations for recording VEPs.

Various preanesthetic medications including phenothiazines, substituted butyrophenones, muscarinic agents, narcotics, and psychomotor stimulants appear to affect the VEP in relation to the physiologic state of the individual. Drugs that enhance the alpha rhythm of the EEG enhance the VEP, with drugs inducing sleep usually causing a degradation of VEPs. Morphine produces no significant effect on the VEP (Corssen & Domino, 1964). Atropine has no significant effect on the VEP, with scopolamine bromide enhancing the VEP responses. The effects of differing concentrations of halothane on the VEP have been variable.

General anesthetics also have variable effects on the VEP. Nitrous oxide has effects ranging from none to occasional enhancement of the VEP (Domino, 1967). Diethyl ether and cyclopropane can depress the VEP. The effects of halothane range from enhancement of later components to no effects (Domino, 1967) to significant increases in the latency of response at 0.5% concentration to abolishment of the VEP at concentrations of 1% (Schramm, Cedzich, Fahlbusch, Mokrusch, & Hochstetter, 1986; Wang, Costa e Silva, Symon, & Jewkes, 1985). Thiamyl sodium effects are dose dependent. At low concentrations, enhancement of the VEP is observed, at intermediate concentrations reductions in the early components and enhancement of the late components are observed, and at high concentrations the response is abolished.

Comparatively few studies have assessed the effect of drugs on PVEPs. Some sedative agents have been used in recording PVEPs. Reliable PVEPs have been recorded in children under chloral hydrate sedation (Wright et al., 1986) which suggests the PVEP may be less susceptible than the FVEP to sedative agents. Russ, Kling, Loesevitz, and Hempelmann (1984) and Burrows, Hillier, McLeod, Iron, and Taylor (1990) have found correlation between VEPs and body temperature. Generally, as body temperature decreases, latencies increase and amplitudes decrease.

PRIOR STUDIES USING VEPs IN IOM

Studies demonstrating the benefits of using visual evoked potentials during intraoperative studies have mainly consisted of case reports:

1. Albright and Sclabassi (1985) were able to record FVEPs consistently during chiasmal glioma surgery in two patients. They found an FVEP could be recorded while an ultrasonic surgical aspirator was used to resect a chiasmal glioma. A strobe light stimulator was used for providing stimulation.

2. Feinsod, Selhorst, Hoyt, and Wilson (1976) found that an FVEP allowed the surgical team to observe a return of function of the optic nerve in a case with a pituitary tumor compressing the optic nerve. They used a contact lens stimulation system to elicit the FVEPs.

3. In six parasellar surgical interventions, Wilson et al. (1976) found intraoperative LED-VEPs correlated with postoperative vision in four cases, one response did not change although vision improved, and one case resulted in an improvement in the LED-VEP with a concomitant loss in vision. An LED goggle stimulation system was used to record the FVEPs.

4. Keenan, Taylor, Coles, Prieur, and Burrows (1987) used FVEPs to monitor visual function in two groups of children during surgery for congenital cardiac abnormalities. Visual system dysfunction is commonly found in cardiovascular surgery (Myendorf, 1982; Smith & Cross, 1982). One group remained on continuous cardiopulmonary bypass, with the other group cooled to lower temperatures before the induction of circulatory stasis and venous exsanguination. They found less impairment in FVEPs in the continuous cardiopulmonary bypass group. They concluded that the FVEP appeared to be useful as an objective measure of short-term effects of cardiopulmonary procedures on neurophysiological function.

LIMITATIONS

Large prospective studies using intraoperative VEPs to predict visual outcome have generally demonstrated little success (Allen, Starr, & Nudleman, 1981; Cedzich, Schramm, Mengledoht, & Fahlbusch, 1988; Raduzens, 1982). Cedzich et al. (1988) reviewed 35 patients with various neurosurgical interventions, including 3 lesions of the orbit, 25 perisellar tumors, 4 intraventricular tumors, 2 occipital tumors, and 1 pineal tumor. Twenty-five patients showed a loss in VEP during surgery. Twenty patients had visual function measured postoperatively, with 12 showing an improvement in acuity, 7 showing no change in acuity, and 1 showing a mild loss in acuity from 20/50 to 20/60.

In another large study (N = 71 patients) Raudzens (1982) found that 81% of subjects had a transient change in the VEP during surgery, 13% had results that could not be interpreted because of artifacts, and 6% showed permanent VEP changes. Raudzens (1982) made no attempt to define a significant change. Allen et al. (1981) reported 68% transient changes in VEP and 12% artifact. A large number of false positives were observed (5/71 patients), with a normal VEP recorded, but a decrease in visual acuity.

Complete absence of FVEPs has been found in patients with normal visual acuity, while preservation of the FVEP did not rule out poor visual outcome (Allen et al., 1981; Raudzens, 1982).

False negative results might be easily explained from technical difficulties, including movement of electrodes, line transients, and uncontrolled stimulation conditions. In addition, preexisting visual abnormalities, anesthetic level, or body temperature may contribute to decrements in VEPs without associated visual loss.

False positives are a serious problem associated with VEPs during IOM. Bodis-Wollner, Atkin, Raab, and Wolkstein (1977) found normal FVEPs in a blind patient. Imaging studies found damage in Brodmann's areas 18 and 19. PVEPs could only be recorded to low spatial frequencies. Celesia, Archer, Kuroiwa, and Goldfader (1972) also reported similar findings in a cortically blind patient.

FUTURE DIRECTIONS

The literature review reveals:

1. Specialized recordings such as the use of a brow ERG (Gouras & MacKay, 1988) to record early postchiasmatic responses may be more useful in assessing the parasellar region, because the VEP reflects function of the entire posterior visual pathway, including striate and extrastriate cortex. Inherent noise in the system might be reduced by only recording from areas of interest. In addition, for applications of electrodiagnostic testing in cardiovascular surgery, the ERG might be more useful. The a/b wave ratio of the flash ERG has been shown to be of benefit in assessing other retinal vascular abnormalities.

2. It is clear that FVEPs have not resulted in diagnostically useful information, because of the high percentages of false positive and negative responses. Use of patterned stimuli may be useful, although Bagoloni, Penne, Fonda, & Mazzetti (1979) found no correlation between PVEPs and visual acuity in four patients. It is clear that the PVEP yields better diagnostic information regarding acuity than the FVEP in nonsurgical monitoring (Hughs, Fino, & Sagnon 1984; Norcia & Tyler, 1985; Wright et al., 1986).

3. One technique that has been used in VEP recording in nonsurgical applications that might be of benefit during surgery is the use of "sweep" techniques. Sweep techniques allow one to get rapid estimates of visual acuity in children (usually in less than 10 sec) by presenting stimuli that are varying in spatial frequency and that are time-locked to the recording apparatus (Norcia & Tyler, 1985).

4. Accessibility to the primary visual pathway might be useful during intraoperative monitoring. The retina, especially the photoreceptor layer, is metabolically active and is susceptible to anoxic damage. The ERG may be useful in assessing retinal damage during surgery (Miyake, Yagasaki, & Horiguchi, 1991). The optic nerve head is sensitive to damage from changes in pressure: acute increases in either intraocular pressure or in intracranial pressure can damage the ganglion cell axons exiting at the nerve head.

SUMMARY

The VEP is easily measured clinically; however, there is a large amount of intrasubject and intersubject variability. The FVEP appears to be susceptible to a number of external perturbations including temperature and preanesthetic and general anesthetic agents. Further work is needed to improve recording VEPs during surgery.

ACKNOWLEDGMENTS

The comments of Thomas Ogden, M.D., Ph.D. and Stephen Russell, M.D. were greatly appreciated.

REFERENCES

Albright, A. L., & Sclabassi, R. J. (1985). Cavitron ultrasonic surgical aspirator and visual evoked potential monitoring for chiasmal gliomas in children. *Journal of Neurosurgery, 63,* 138–140.

Allen, A., Starr, A., & Nudleman, K. (1981). Assessment of sensory function in the operating room utilizing cerebral evoked potentials: A study of 56 surgically anesthetized patients. *Clinical Neurosurgery, 28,* 457–481.

Bagolini, B. A., Penne, A., Fonda, S., & Mazzetti, A. (1979). Pattern visual evoked potentials in general anesthesia. *Archiv fuer Klinische und Experimentelle Ophthalmologie, 209,* 231–238.

Bassi, C. J., & Lehmkuhle, S. (1990). Clinical implications of parallel visual pathways. *Journal of the American Optometric Association, 61,* 98–110.

Bodis-Wollner, I., Atkin, A., Raab, W., & Wolkstein, M. (1977). Visual association cortex and vision in man. Pattern vision in a blind boy. *Science, 198,* 639–640.

Burrows, F. A., Hillier, S. C., McLeod, M. E., Iron, K. S., & Taylor, M. J. (1990). Anterior fontanel pressure and visual evoked potentials in neonates and infants undergoing profound hypothermic circulatory arrest. *Anesthesiology, 73,* 632–636.

Carr, R. E., & Siegel, I. M. (1990). *Electrodiagnostic testing of the visual system: A clinical guide.* Philadelphia, F. A. Davis Company.

Cedzich, C., Schramm, J., Mengledoht, C. F., & Fahlbusch, R. (1988). Factors that limit the use of flash evoked potentials for surgical monitoring. *Electroencephalography and Clinical Neurophysiology, 71,* 142–148.

Celesia, G. G., Archer, C. R., Kuroiwa, Y., & Goldfader, P. R. (1972). Visual function of the extrageniculo-calcarine system in man. *Archives of Neurology, 37,* 704–706.

Clark, D. L., & Rosner, B. S. (1973). Neurophysiologic effect of general anesthetics. 1. The electroencephalogram and sensory evoked responses. *Anesthesiology, 38,* 564–582.

Corssen, G., & Domino, E. F. (1964). Visually evoked potentials in man: A method for measuring cerebral effects of preanesthetic medication. *Anesthesiology, 25,* 330–337.

DeYoe, E. A., & VanEssen, D. C. (1988). Concurrent processing streams in monkey visual cortex. *Trends in Neuroscience, 11,* 219–26.

Domino, E. F. (1967). Effects of preanesthetic and anesthetic drugs on visually evoked responses. *Anesthesiology, 28,* 184–191.

Evoked Potentials Committee (1987). American Electroencephalographic Society guidelines for intraoperative monitoring of sensory evoked potentials. *Journal of Clinical Neurophysiology, 4,* 397–416.

Fahlbusch, R. (1981). Optic nerve compression by pituitary adenomas. In M. Samii & P. J. Jannetta (Eds.), *The cranial nerves* (pp. 140–147). New York, Springer-Verlag.

Feinsod, M., Selhorst, J. B., Hoyt, W. F., & Wilson, C.B., (1976). *Journal of Neurosurgery, 44,* 29–31.

Gouras, P. & MacKay, C. J. (1988). Detecting early postchiasmal visually evoked responses. *Clinical Vision Science, 3,* 119–124.

Grundy, B. L. (1982). Monitoring of sensory evoked potentials during neurosurgical operations: Methods and applications. *Neurosurgery, 11,* 556–575.

Hacke, W. (1985). Neuromonitoring. *Journal of Neurology, 232,* 125–133.

Halliday, A. M., Barret, S., Caroll, W. M., & Kriss, S. (1982). Problems in defining normal limits of visual evoked potential. In J. Courjon, F. M. Mauguiere, and M. Revol (Eds.), *Clinical applications of evoked potentials in neurology* (pp. 1–9). New York: Raven Press.

Harding, G. F. A., Smith, V. H., & Yorke, H. C. (1987). A contact lens stimulator for surgical monitoring. *Electroencephalography and Clinical Neurophysiology, 66,* 322–328.

Horwitz, N. H., & Rizzoli, H. V. (1982). Postoperative complications of intracranial neurological surgery (pp. 95–141). Baltimore: Williams and Wilkins.

Hughs, J. R., Fino, J., & Sagnon, L. (1984). A comparison of flash and pattern evoked potentials in patients with demyelinating disease and in normal controls. In R. H. Nodar & B. Colin (Eds.), *Evoked potentials II* (pp. 302–309). Boston: Butterworth Publishers.

Kaas J. H. (1986). The structural basis for information processing the primate visual system. In J. D. Pettigrew, K. J. Sanderson, & W. R. Levick (Eds.), *Visual neuroscience* (pp. 302–309). New York: Cambridge University Press.

Keenan, N. K., Taylor, M. J., Coles, J. G., Prieur, B. J., & Burrows, F. A. (1987). The use of VEPs for CNS monitoring during continuous cardiopulmonary bypass and circulatory arrest. *Electroencephalography and Clinical Neurophysiology, 68,* 241–246.

Miyake, Y., Yagasaki, K., & Horiguchi, M. (1991). Electroretinographic monitoring of retinal function during eye surgery. *Archives of Ophthalmology, 109,* 1123–1126.

Myendorf, R. (1982). Psychopatho-ophthalmology, gnostic disorders and psychosis in cardiac surgery. *Archiv fuer Psychiatrie und Nervenkrankheiten, 232,* 119–125.

Norcia, A. M., & Tyler, C. W. (1985). Spatial frequency sweep VEP: Visual acuity during the first year of life. *Vision Research, 25,* 1399–1408.

Pollock, V. E., Schneifer, L. S., Chui, H. C., Henderson, V., Zemansky, M., & Sloane, R. B. (1989). Visual evoked potentials in dementia: A meta-analysis and empirical study of Alzheimer's disease patients. *Biological Psychiatry, 25,* 1003–1013.

Raduzens, P. A. (1982). Intraoperative monitoring of evoked potentials. *Annals of the New York Academy of Science, 82,* 308–326.

Regan, D. (1989). *Human brain electrophysiology.* New York: Elsevier.

Russ, W., Kling, D., Loesevitx, A., & Hempelmann, G. (1984). Effect of hypothermia on visual evoked potentials (VEP) in humans. *Anesthesiology, 61,* 207–210.

Sadun, A. A. (1986). Neuroanatomy of the human visual system: Part I Retinal projection to the LGN and pretectum as demonstrated with a new method. *Neuro-ophthalmology, 6,* 353–361.

Sadun, A. A., Johnson, B. M., & Schaechter, J. (1986). Neuroanatomy of the human visual system: Part III Three retinal projections to the hypothalamus. *Neuro-ophthalmology, 6,* 371–379.

Sadun, A. A., Johnson, B.M., & Smith, L. E. H. (1986). Neuroanatomy of the human visual system: Part II Retinal projection to the superior colliculus and pulvinar. *Neuro-ophthalmology, 6,* 363–370.

Schramm, J., Cedzich, C., Fahlbusch, R., Mokrusch, T., & Hochstetter, H. (1986). Intraoperative monitoring of evoked potentials for surgery in and around the third ventricle and the brain stem. In M. Samii (Ed.), *Surgery in and around the brain stem and third ventricle: Anatomy, pathology, neurophysiology, diagnosis, treatment* (pp. 154–160). Berlin: Springer-Verlag.

Smith, J. L., & Cross, S. A. (1983). Occipital lobe infarction after open heart surgery. *Journal of Clinical Neuro-ophthalmology, 3,* 23–30.

Sokol, S. (1976). Visually evoked potentials: Theory, techniques and clinical applications. *Survey of Ophthalmology, 21,* 18–44.

Wang, A. D-J, Costa e Silva, I., Symon, L., & Jewkes D. (1985). The effect of halothane on somatosensory and flash visual evoked potentials during operations. *Neurological Research, 7,* 58–62.

Wilson, W. B., Kirsch, W. M., Neville, H., Stears, J., Feinsod, M., & Lehman, A. W. (1976). Monitoring of visual function during parasellar surgery. *Surgical Neurology, 5,* 323–329.

Wright, J. E., Arden, G., & Jones, B. R. (1973). Continuous monitoring of the visually evoked response during intra-orbital surgery. *Transactions of the Ophthalmological Society, United Kingdom, 93,* 311–324.

Wright, K. W., Eriksen, J., Shors, T. J., & Ary J. P. (1986). Recording pattern visual evoked potentials under chloryl hydrate sedation. *Archives of Ophthalmology, 104,* 718–721.

CHAPTER 2

MONITORING THE EXTRAOCULAR NERVES

AUKSE E. BANKAITIS, M.A.
ROBERT W. KEITH, Ph.D.

Elevated awareness of the benefits of neurophysiological intraoperative monitoring within the medical profession has led to the increased demand for such services. Since 1988, the number of orthopedic and neurosurgical cases monitored by the division of Intraoperative Monitoring at the University of Cincinnati Medical Center has increased by 440%. Part of the reason for such widespread progress stems from the accumulation of evidence on the efficacy of intraoperative monitoring in reducing postoperative neurologic deficits (Moller, 1992). The increased demand for neurophysiological intraoperative monitoring has also broadened the application of more traditional monitoring techniques (Keith & Bankaitis, 1993). For example, the auditory brainstem response (ABR) continues as a key method for attaining serviceable hearing during acoustic tumor removal (Lenarz & Ernst, 1992), and the application of this technique has also been effective for monitoring brainstem function during cerebral aneurysm surgery and microvascular decompression for the treatment of trigeminal neuralgia and hemifacial spasm (Keith & Bankaitis, 1993; Lenarz & Ernst, 1992; Manninen, Cuillerier, Nantau, & Gelb, 1992; Moller & Moller, 1989; Mori, Takahashi, Yanase, & Suzuki, 1990; Sindou,

Fobe, Ciriano, & Fischer, 1992). Similarly, requests for intraoperative cranial nerve monitoring have increased beyond requests for facial and auditory nerves to include observation of other cranial nerves. With the exception of electrode placement, the basic technique involved in monitoring the extraocular nerves, the innervators of the eye muscles, stems from the same principles applied during facial nerve monitoring. One of the biggest obstacles involved in monitoring the extraocular nerves is the lack of familiarization with the anatomy of oculomotor (III), trochlear (IV), and abducens (VI) cranial nerves. To effectively execute intraoperative monitoring, familiarization with fundamental anatomy is essential. A major portion of this chapter covers anatomic aspects of the oculomotor system.

THE OCULOMOTOR SYSTEM

Visual detection of objects relies on a visual angle covering approximately 200°. Objects are best seen with the fovea, a small patch of densely packed cones located at the center of each retina (Barber & Stockwell, 1980; Goldberg, Eggers, & Gouras, 1991). The fovea is a very small area in the center of the retina. It is less than 1 mm in diameter. Because of the poor resolving power of the retina, the oculomotor system must efficiently coordinate the movement of both eyes onto a chosen target (Barber & Stockwell, 1980). Once the desired visual target is on the fovea, the oculomotor system functions to maintain eye position on the visual target (Goldberg, Eggers, & Gouras, 1991).

To change and maintain visual fixation in a precise and synchronized fashion, higher centers within the cortex and brainstem regulate extraocular muscle movement by the coordinated activity of three motor cranial nerves (Wilson-Pauwels, Akesson, & Stewart, 1988). The oculomotor (CN III), trochlear (CN IV), and abducens (CN VI) nerves are ultimately responsible for innervating the extraocular muscles. Collectively, this triad of cranial nerves is interchangeably referred to as either the extraocular nerves or oculomotor nerves. To avoid confusion with individual reference to CN III (the oculomotor nerve), the term extraocular nerves will be used to refer collectively to CN III, IV, and VI.

THE ORBIT

The orbit is a bony walled cavity, or socket, in which both eyes develop separately. A pattern of bones, namely the maxilla and palatine, the frontal, sphenoid, zygomatic, ethmoid, and lacrimal, form the orbital wall (Wolff, 1976). Lined with a tough membrane, or periosteum, the orbit contains an additional layer of fat. This structural orbit design cushions and protects the eyes from external injury.

The orbit also houses essential muscles, nerves, and vessels. The extraocular nerves, the ophthalmic branch of the trigeminal nerve (CN V), and the ophthalmic vein extend through the superior orbital fissure. In addition, the optic nerve extends from the back of the eye through a small opening in the orbit, the optic foramen (Abrahamson, 1972). Damage to the orbital wall can lead to serious complications, including infection of the orbital cavity or ocular misalignment (Goldberg, 1991).

CRANIAL NERVE III

Of the three extraocular nerves, CN III is the most complex. Not only does it innervate four of the six extraocular muscles, but it bilaterally supplies the levator palpebrae superioris, the elevator of the upper eyelids. In contrast to the trochlear and abducens nerves, CN III contains axons of autonomic preganglionic neurons (Martin, 1989), providing presynaptic parasympathetic outflow to the ciliary and sphincter muscles of the iris. As a result of such numerous innervations, complete loss of oculomotor function typically results in functional blindness of the affected eye (Moller, 1988).

Positioned within the midbrain, a pair of cell masses located at the level of the superior colliculus just below the floor of the third ventricle comprise the nucleus of CN III. Dorsal to the anterior portion of the oculomotor nucleus lies the Edinger-Westphal nucleus, the visceral motor center responsible for innervating the constrictor pupillae and the ciliary muscles (Wilson-Pauwels, Akesson, & Stewart, 1988).

Fibers of the oculomotor nerve leave the nuclear complex to course ventrally through the red nucleus. Exiting the brainstem through the medial portion of each cerebral peduncle, the nerve emerges from the interpeduncular fossa to pass between the posterior cerebral and superior cerebellar arteries. It continues to travel lateral and parallel with the posterior communicating artery of the circle of Willis. As it pierces the dura, CN III enters the cavernous sinus and travels along the lateral wall to eventually enter the orbit of the eye. Entering the orbit through the superior orbital fissure, the nerve branches into a superior and inferior division, forming multiple ramifications that innervate individual muscles (Feldon & Burde, 1992; Sacks, 1984).

CRANIAL NERVE IV

The nucleus of the trochlear nerve (CN IV) originates within the tegmentum of the midbrain at the level of the inferior colliculus. Practically continuous with the caudal portion of the oculomotor nucleus, the trochlear nucleus indents the dorsal surface of a bidirectional fiber tract called the medial longitudinal fasciculus (MLF) (Feldon & Burde, 1992). Axons of the trochlear motor neurons course caudally in the periaqueductal gray along the lateral margin of the cerebral aqueduct and fourth ventricle.

Two unique anatomical features of the trochlear nerve deserve mention. Dorsal to the cerebral aqueduct at the junction of the pons and midbrain lies the isthmus, a constriction in the diameter of the brainstem (Martin, 1989). Unlike all other cranial nerves, prior to exiting the brainstem, the axons of the trochlear nerve cross midline within the isthmus of the pons. Secondly, the trochlear nerve exits the midbrain from the dorsal surface. The complete decussation and the dorsal emergence of the trochlear nerve contribute to its characteristically long intracranial course.

Once the nerve exits the brainstem, it courses anterior and ventral in the subarachnoid space, around the cerebral peduncles (basis pedunculi) to pierce the dura and enters the cavernous sinus. As it travels along the lateral wall of the sinus, the trochlear nerve remains ventral to the oculomotor nerve. Entering the orbit through the superior orbital fissure, the trochlear nerve divides into three branches and terminates on the superior oblique muscle.

CRANIAL NERVE VI

The abducens nucleus lies in the tegmental portion of the caudal pons just ventral to the floor of the fourth ventricle. Medial to the nucleus lie the motor fibers of the facial nerve that loop around the dorsal aspect of the abducens nucleus. The nature of this course creates a bulge in the floor of the fourth ventricle known as the facial colliculus.

The sixth nerve fibers course ventrally through the pons to emerge at its base at the pontomedullary junction. The nerve then turns rostrally and laterally in the subarachnoid space, crossing over the tip of the petrous portion of the temporal bone. As the nerve penetrates the dura, it enters the cavernous sinus and runs medial to cranial nerves III, IV, and V and near the carotid artery. Reaching the orbit via the superior orbital fissure, the nerve supplies the lateral rectus muscle.

EXTRAOCULAR MUSCLES

There are six extrinsic muscles of the eye: the medial rectus, inferior rectus, superior rectus, lateral rectus, superior oblique and inferior oblique. All of the extraocular muscles insert into the sclera, the tough fibrous coating of the eye, via collagenous tendons that eventually become indistinguishable from the sclera (Wolff, 1976). In addition, each extraocular muscle connects to the nasal aspect of the orbit. The extraocular muscles do not attach to the temporal wall of the orbit (Goldberg, 1991).

EXTRAOCULAR MUSCLES INNERVATED BY CRANIAL NERVE III

Reaching the orbit, the oculomotor nerve branches into an inferior and superior division. The inferior division supplies the ipsilateral medial and inferior recti muscles and the ipsilateral inferior oblique muscle. The medial rectus, the largest of the extraocular muscles, arises on the inner side of the lower optic foramen just below the ophthalmic artery (Dyer & Lee, 1984). As it travels anteriorly, it hugs the medial orbital wall and inserts into the sclera approximately 5.3 mm from the limbus, the junction of the cornea and sclera (Goldberg, 1991). The medial rectus is a pure adductor and is responsible for moving the eye nasally.

The inferior rectus muscle, the shortest of all four recti muscles, arises below the optic foramen and temporarily courses within the orbit. On reaching the floor of the orbit, the inferior rectus muscle runs above the inferior oblique and inserts 6.8 mm from the limbus. This muscle primarily depresses the abducted eye, aids in the adduction, and extorts the eye when it is turned inward (Dyer & Lee, 1984). The inferior oblique arises from the periosteum of the orbital floor and courses laterally and posteriorly between the inferior rectus and the floor of the orbit (Dyer & Lee, 1984). This muscle elevates the eye when it is already abducted.

The superior motor fibers of the oculomotor nerve ascend laterally, innervating the ipsilateral superior rectus and the levator palpebrae superioris muscles bilaterally. As with all the recti muscles, the superior rectus arises from the upper portion of a short tendinous ring know as the annulus of Zinn (Wolff, 1976). The primary action of the superior rectus involves elevation of the eye, an action which increases as the eye turns laterally. In addition, this muscle also adducts and intorts the eye (Dyer & Lee, 1984).

The levator palpebrae superioris arises from the undersurface of the lesser wing of the sphenoid bone dorsal and anterior to the optic foramen. Coursing anteriorly below the roof of the orbit, it eventually attaches to the skin of the upper eyelid (Wolff, 1976) to elevate the eyelid. Additional motor fibers from the Edinger-Westphal nucleus supply the sphincter muscles of the iris and ciliary muscles of the lens, contributing to the capability of the oculomotor nerve to control pupil constriction and lens shape.

EXTRAOCULAR MUSCLE INNERVATED
BY CRANIAL NERVE IV

The longest and thinnest of all the extraocular muscles, the superior oblique is innervated by the contralateral trochlear nucleus. Originating from the lesser wing of the sphenoid bone, the superior oblique courses anteriorly until it reaches the trochlea, a U-shaped cartilaginous extension of the frontal bone. As it runs through the trochlea, the superior oblique bends sharply and courses back along the upper surface of the globe before attaching to the lateral aspect of the sclera (Carl, 1993). The primary action of the superior oblique is to depress an already adducted eye.

EXTRAOCULAR MUSCLES INNERVATED
BY CRANIAL NERVE VI

The lateral rectus muscle extends anteriorly on the temporal side of the globe and inserts about 7 mm from the limbus via a long thin tendon. In contrast to the medial rectus muscle, the abducens nerve innervates the lateral rectus muscle, which abducts the eye. Although the medial and lateral recti muscles are responsible for shifting the axis of vision in opposite directions, the two muscles work together to move the eyes along the horizontal plane. For instance, as both eyes shift from center to lateral gaze, higher centers execute simultaneous contraction of the ipsilateral lateral rectus and the contralateral medial rectus muscles. A general understanding of higher centers is necessary to fully appreciate implications of various oculomotor deficits.

HIGHER CENTERS OF OCULOMOTOR SYSTEM

Two cortical regions, the parieto-occipital eye field and frontal eye field, are responsible for controlling eye movements. Located at the juncture of the parietal and occipital lobes, the parieto-occipital eye field sends poorly defined pathways to the extraocular neurons to initiate bilateral contraction of the medial recti muscles, resulting in the movement of both eyes toward midline (convergence). Rostral to the supplementary motor and premotor cortex, pathways projecting from the frontal eye field (Brodmann's area 8) reach various brainstem nuclear regions, two of which include the rostral interstitial nucleus of the medial longitudinal fasciculus (MLF) and the paramedian pontine reticular formation (PPRF) (Martin, 1989).

The rostral interstitial nucleus of the MLF is a localized region within the tegmental area of the midbrain rostral to the oculomotor complex. Presumably, this nucleus not only controls vertical eye movements (Buttner, Buttner-Ennever, & Henn, 1977), but plays a key role in the coordination of conjugate eye movements (Martin, 1989) through its connection with the MLF. The MLF is a bidirectional, paired fiber tract extending from the reticular substance of the midbrain and thalamus to the anterior horn cells of the cervical spinal cord (Evinger, Fuchs, & Baker, 1977; Feldon & Burde, 1992; Honrubia & Hoffman, 1993; Maciewicz & Spencer, 1977). It centrally connects the extraocular nuclei with each other as well as with the PPRF.

Receiving input mainly from the interstitial nucleus of the MLF and superior colliculus, the PPRF is the supranuclear center for the control of conjugate eye movements (Feldon & Burde, 1992). On receiving input from these central nervous system centers, the PPRF projects directly back to the abducens nucleus and interstitial nucleus of the MLF (Buttner, Buttner-Ennever, & Henn, 1977) to integrate horizontal and vertical components of coordinated eye movements (Carpenter, 1985).

To produce rapid eye movements the extraocular muscles on both sides must act precisely and synergistically (Carpenter, 1985). Initiation of saccadic eye movements requires a burst of high frequency discharge to agonist muscles with a corresponding period of inhibition of the antagonist muscles (Ingram, Wilson, Arnold, & Dally, 1986; Jacobson, Sandberg, Effron, & Berson, 1979). These required timing signals are generated by the PPRF (Boothe, Tigges, & Wilson, 1990; Carpenter, 1985; Nolte, 1988). For both eyes to voluntarily look rapidly to the left, the right frontal eye field issues a command to the left PPRF, which sends impulses to the ipsilateral abducens nucleus to initiate contraction of the left lateral rectus muscle via the abducens nerve. The left PPRF simultaneously coordinates the interneurons of the left abducens nucleus, whose axons cross midline to the contralateral MLF, to influence the contraction of the right medial rectus muscle by the right oculomotor nucleus and nerve (Nolte, 1988).

LESIONS OF CN III, IV, AND VI

Damage to specific structures within the oculomotor system is often associated with a particular site of lesion. Although these associations are convenient in terms of localization, it is important to distinguish eye movement deficits resulting from a lesion of an extraocular nerve from those caused by an extraocular nucleus lesion.

Extraocular nerve lesions cause characteristic abnormalities of the eye. For example, damage to the oculomotor nerve may cause ipsilateral paralysis or weakness of the respective extraocular muscles. This results in abduction of the eye (lateral strabismus), with the inability to turn the eye medially or vertically; dilation of the pupil (mydriasis); drooping of the upper eyelid (ptosis); and/or double vision (diplopia). A lesion of the trochlear nerve may result in paralysis or weakness in downward and lateral gaze. An injured abducens nerve may result in medial strabismus as the lateral rectus muscle can no longer receive input from the brain to pull the eye laterally from midline. As a result, the medial rectus muscle will continue to receive input from the brain to contract and, in doing so, pull the eye medially.

Damage to the nucleus may also result in identifiable deficits in and around the eye; however, additional dysfunction may also be present. In contrast to an isolated abducens nerve lesion, which typically results in medial strabismus, damage to the abducens nucleus may hamper medial movement of the contralateral eye. A damaged abducens nucleus will not be able to provide the necessary input to the abducens nerve for contraction of the lateral rectus muscle. Damage to only one abducens nucleus causes a loss of all horizontal eye movements to the ipsilateral side (Nolte, 1988). This deficit in lateral gaze is referred to as lateral gaze palsy.

Common causes of extraocular cranial nerve palsies include ischemic lesions, particularly in patients who are diabetic (Carl, 1993). Aneurysm of the posterior cerebral or superior cerebellar arteries may cause CN III problems, because the nerve emerges between both arteries (Wilson-Pauwels, Akesson, & Stewart, 1988). The most common cause of trochlear nerve palsy is head trauma (Carl, 1993). The trochlear nerve (CN IV) is also susceptible to inflammatory disease, compression attributable to aneurysm of the posterior cerebral and superior cerebellar arteries, and cavernous sinus or superior orbital fissure lesions (Wilson-Pauwels, Akesson, & Stewart, 1988). Similarly, the abducens nerve is commonly affected by trauma, iatrogenic injury, or increased intracranial pressure (Carl, 1993).

INTRAOPERATIVE MONITORING TECHNIQUE

Regardless of the specific nerve to be monitored, the goals of cranial nerve monitoring are threefold: (1) to assist in early nerve identification, (2) to increase the likelihood of neural preservation by minimizing trauma, and (3) to assess neural integrity following dissection (Kartush, 1989). Monitoring one or any combination of the three oculomotor nerves is appropriate during surgical cases that may jeopardize functional integrity of the nerves. In our experience, these nerves have been monitored during surgical cases involving exploration of brainstem arterial venous malformations (AVM), lesions of the cavernous sinus, removal of a meningioma involving the petrous ridge, holocavernous lesion involving the carotid artery, and removal of middle fossa infiltrating meningioma.

EQUIPMENT

Although a number of devices are available to monitor cranial nerve EMG activity, we use the Nerve Integrity Monitor-2 (NIM-2, Xomed-Treace, Inc., Jacksonville, Florida; Figure 2-1).

One advantage of this system is that it simultaneously provides visual and auditory feedback of electromyographic activity and allows immediate interpretation of responses within the context of the surgical events (Kartush, 1989). In addition, a muting system automatically eliminates electrical artifact during the operative procedure as a result of extensive use of electrocautery equipment (Bankaitis & Keith, 1993). Evoked potential equipment can also be used to monitor cranial nerve function. For simultaneous monitoring of several cranial nerves, we prefer a multiple channel EMG recording system, such as the Nerve Integrity Monitor (NIM-2).

ANESTHESIA

Any time cranial nerve function is monitored, long-acting muscle relaxants or neuromuscular blocking agents should be avoided. During initial induction of anesthesia, paralyzing drugs may be utilized during patient preparation. However, once the structures to be monitored are surgically approached, paralyzing drug effects must be reversed. Even low doses of muscle relaxants that do not effect nerve responses from direct electrical stimulation may compromise electromyography (EMG). As a result, small amplitude responses associated with mechanical manipulations in the presence of low level neuromuscular blocking agents may be undetectable (Kartush & Bouchard, 1992).

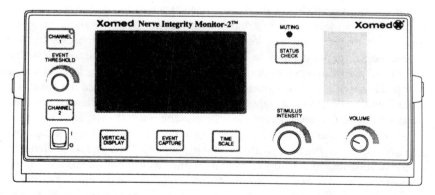

FIGURE 2-1. Front panel of the Nerve Integrity Monitor-2 (NIM-2, Xomed-Treace, Inc., Jacksonville, Florida). Touch pads on the right side of the device allow for simultaneous monitoring of up to two channels.

ELECTRODES

Although various types of electrodes are available, subdermal needle electrodes are preferred for intraoperative monitoring of the extraocular nerves. Needle electrodes permit rapid and secure placement (Kartush & Bouchard, 1992). In contrast to surface electrodes applied with electrode paste, the impedance of needle electrodes does not change over time. These are necessary advantages, because limited patient preparation time and extended recording sessions are more typical of most surgical cases that incorporate intraoperative monitoring.

Once the patient is anesthetized, needle electrodes are inserted intramuscularly. To monitor CN III, IV, and VI, a needle electrode is inserted in or near the inferior rectus, superior oblique, and lateral rectus muscles, respectively. Needle electrodes can be placed in or near these muscles percutaneously; it is not necessary to penetrate the extraocular muscles with the needle electrode. They state that electrodes placed within the vicinity of the muscle will produce sufficient EMG response amplitudes for monitoring. In cases with CN VI and CN VII simultaneously monitored, we place a hook wire electrode just inside the lateral orbit near the lateral rectus muscle to monitor the abducens nerve. Because of the close proximity of the lateral rectus to the orbicularis oculi muscles, problems of response interpretation may arise regarding whether the response is a result of lateral rectus muscle versus orbicularis oris muscle activity. Extreme caution is necessary when inserting needle electrodes within the vicinity of the extraocular muscles to avoid injury to the globe of the eye. Once the active needle electrode is inserted near the extraocular muscle, the reference electrode should be inserted on the opposite side of the head. Note that only a reference electrode is required despite simultaneous monitoring of more than one extraocular nerve (Figure 2–2).

Once electrodes are inserted into the proper response sites, functional electrode integrity must be verified. As with any electrophysiological test, obtaining the lowest possible electrode impedances is desirable (less than 5,000 ohms). Impedances should be balanced resulting in inter-electrode impedances of less than 1,000 ohms. These standards reduce the "antenna-like" quality of electrode input wires because higher impedances are more susceptible to the detection of electromagnetic noise (Prass, 1992).

Once normal electrode impedances have been achieved, we further verify electrode function with a "touch" or "tap" test (Beck & Benecke, 1990). Touching or tapping the vicinity of the electrode response area should register an audible and visual response from and on the oscilloscopic display of the NIM-2. This simple procedure confirms proper operation of the recording equipment.

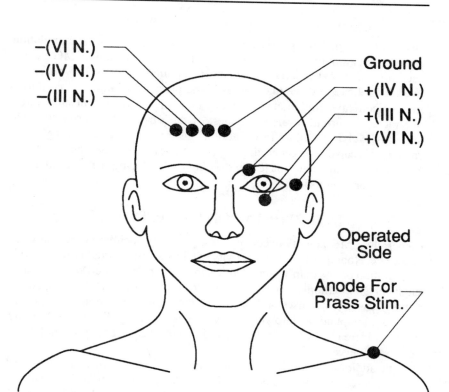

FIGURE 2–2. A needle electrode inserted near the inferior rectus, superior oblique, and lateral rectus muscles is necessary to monitor CN III, IV, and VI, respectively. At least one electrode should be inserted in the forehead on the opposite side of the head to serve as a reference.

STIMULATING PROBES

There are two types of stimulating probes available: monopolar and bipolar. Both types are suitable for stimulating nerve fibers intracranially, however, monopolar stimulation is suitable for mapping the general vicinity of the nerve, with bipolar stimulation much more selective, as it reduces the incidence of false-positive errors from current jumps (Kartush & Bouchard, 1992). One difficulty with bipolar stimulation is the possibility of body fluids shunting the current across the tip of the probe, making the stimulator probe ineffective. Care must be taken to keep a bipolar stimulating probe clean and dry.

Regardless of the type of probe used, the NIM-2 allows manual adjustment of the current stimulus to be delivered through the stimulating probe.

In the absence of established safety limitations for cranial nerve stimulation, the smallest amount of stimulus necessary to elicit a detectable EMG event is recommended. We initially set the current stimulus levels at 0.05 mA; however, identification of cranial nerves in the presence of tumor mass during direct electrical stimulation may require higher levels of current stimulation. We increase current levels on request of the surgeon and strive to avoid stimulus levels exceeding 1 mA. Caution must be used when operating equipment that is capable of generating high current levels. The best guide is to use minimum stimulus current levels capable of producing a sufficient EMG response for monitoring.

INTERPRETATION OF RESPONSES

Generally, EMG activity occurring during surgery is either nonrepetitive or repetitive. Nonrepetitive EMG activity exhibits a "burst" quality with a typical duration of less than 1 second and is most often associated with brief mechanical stimulation of the nerve(s) (Prass & Luders, 1986). Repetitive activity usually increases and decreases with discontinuation of a specific surgical manipulation, implying a causative relationship (Prass, 1992). Long duration increases of background EMG activity may reflect potential damage to the nerve.

In addition to mechanical stimulation, cranial nerve responses may occur as a result of other factors. Drilling adjacent to a nerve may transmit vibrations through surrounding bone inducing what Kartush and Bouchard (1992) refer to as a "drill potential" (Kartush & Bouchard, 1992). A similar response is seen with the use of the cusa. Thermal changes, such as cold water irrigation may evoke responses. It is important to interpret responses within the context of ongoing surgical activities. Synchronous responses, or "pulses," occur as a result of direct electrical stimulation and indicate a functionally intact nerve. Interpretation of cranial nerve responses to direct stimulation is not easy. Although current guidelines regarding cranial nerve monitoring and electrical stimulation are lacking, information about stimulation level and time, duration, and amplitude of responses should be documented throughout an entire surgical procedure. Theoretically, stimulation of an intact nerve proximal and distal to a removed tumor should yield approximately equal response amplitudes; significant decreases in the amplitude of responses elicited from the proximal portion of the nerve may be indicative of postoperative muscle weakness.

COMMUNICATION WITH SURGICAL STAFF

Communication among the entire surgical staff is extremely important. Jacobson and Balzer (1992) state that "intraoperative monitoring is only as good as its weakest link" (Jacobson & Balzer, 1992). Preoperative communication with the entire surgical staff not only confirms procedural expectations, but reduces unnecessary assumptions or confusion that may occur during the surgical procedure. One should never assume that the presence of intraoperative monitoring equipment will be a cue to the anesthesiologist, for example, to avoid using neuromuscular blocking agents.

CASE STUDY 1

A 46-year-old male with a previous unremarkable medical history sustained a head injury on falling backward from a ladder head first. As the patient fell, the occipital area of his head first struck a wooden board then hit the floor. Following an unspecified length of unconsciousness, the patient awoke with numbness of the left hand. Neurophysiological testing revealed an inability to identify objects placed in his left hand. In addition, the patient complained of throbbing headaches, vertigo, eye pain, and CN V parasthesias on the right. Following imaging studies, a diagnosis of a brainstem pontine superior cerebellar peduncle cavernous angioma was made, and the patient was scheduled for surgery. Neurophysiological monitoring of brainstem function was conducted, using the auditory brainstem response (ABR) with insert earphones placed in the right and left ears and response electrodes at Fz references to A1 and A2. In addition, brainstem function was monitored with upper somatosensory cortical evoked potentials (SCEP), with subdermal stimulus electrodes placed near the median nerve at the right and left wrists and response electrodes at C3 and C4 referenced to Cz. To monitor the stability of the evoked potentials below the surgical site, responses were also monitored from the brachial plexus, with electrodes placed just above the clavicle.

Multiple cranial nerves were monitored with needle electrode pairs appropriately placed as follows:

Cranial Nerve	Electrode Placement
Trigeminal (V)	Right temporalis muscle
Abducens (VI)	Lateral orbital rim of both eyes
Facial (VII)	Right orbicularis oris muscle
Vagus (X)	Right vocalis muscle
Accessory (XI)	Right trapezius muscle

To monitor CN VI and X, only one needle electrode was inserted in the appropriate electrode location, with a reference electrode placed in the opposite forehead.

Preincision ABR revealed a normal wave I, III, and V in the left ear with a normal wave I from the right ear, with waves III and V prolonged by 0.4 millisecond. The amplitude of wave V was reduced bilaterally. There was no intraoperative change in the ABR response. Median nerve SCEP were symmetrical and normal prior to surgical incision. Three hours following the initial incision, the SCEP response from the right median nerve severely decreased in amplitude and eventually was completely lost. The left median nerve SCEP remained stable and within normal limits of baseline levels.

Mapping of the cranial nerve nuclei along the floor of the fourth ventricle was done with a stimulus setting of 0.05 uV. The nuclei of CN VI, VII, and X were identified, with response levels of the appropriate muscles ranging from 300 to 1100 uV. We were never able to obtain a response from CN V. No attempt was made to identify the XI nerve.

This patient woke with right side partial paralysis of CN VI and VII that improved postoperatively. The surgeon hypothesized that the temporary paralysis was caused by edema that resolved with time. All other cranial nerves were intact. There was no hemiparesis and the loss of the SCEP from the right median nerve was either a false negative finding or a reflection of intraoperative edema.

CASE STUDY 2

This 55-year-old male with a temporal meningioma underwent a middle fossa anterior petrosectomy for removal of his tumor. Brainstem function was monitored with the auditory brainstem response (ABR) and upper somato-sensory cortical evoked potentials (SCEP). Insert earphones were placed in the right and left ears for ABR testing and the median nerve was stimulated with needle electrode pairs of the right and left wrists. Response electrodes were appropriately placed at C3, C4, A1, A2 referenced to FZ.

In addition, cranial nerves III, IV, V, VI, and VII were monitored. To monitor the extraocular nerves, a needle electrode was placed at the medial canthus (CN III), lateral canthus (CN VI), and inferior to the globe (CN IV), with a reference electrode placed in the opposite forehead. The trigeminal (CN V) and facial (VII) nerves were also monitored, with response needle electrode pairs located in the temporalis and orbicularis oris muscles, respectively.

The ABR remained stable throughout the surgical procedure. The median nerve response from the left was also stable from incision to closure. However, the median nerve response from stimulation on the right side fluctuated and deteriorated. Approximately 7 hours into the procedure, the median nerve response had deteriorated by 50% in amplitude with no change in latency. At 11 hours into the procedure, the response from the median nerve became even poorer and was flat. The response from the left median nerve deteriorated to approximately 50% of the original amplitude. There was no change in the left median nerve response to the end of the case and the right median nerve response never returned. The ABR remained at baseline levels throughout the surgical procedure.

Although direct stimulation of the extraocular nerves was not utilized for this particular case, the spontaneous activity of CN III, IV, and VI was continually monitored from incision to closure. On surgically reaching the brainstem at the level of the rostral pons, distinguishable EMG responses from CN III and IV were recorded and documented as a result of surgical manipulation. At no time was an increase in background EMG activity observed. The responses of both nerves to mechanical stimulation assisted the surgeon in identifying surgical neurostructures, aiding in reducing postoperative morbidity.

SUMMARY

Although the basic principles of facial nerve monitoring apply to the extraocular nerves, the effectiveness and quality of the intraoperative monitoring begins with a thorough understanding of the anatomy of CN III, IV, and VI. Without an anatomical knowledge base, the ability to assist in early nerve identification and preservation is significantly minimized. The provision of cranial nerve monitoring services extends beyond anatomical and technical considerations. Because the integrity of electromyographic activity of any cranial nerve may be readily influenced by numerous extraneous variables, awareness of the affects of such factors, particularly in the area of anesthesia, must be considered. In addition, the maintenance of constant communication between the entire surgical staff throughout the entirety of surgical procedures is equally essential.

REFERENCES

Abrahamson, I. (1972). *Know your eyes.* New York: Medcom Press.

Bankaitis, A., & Keith, R. (1993). Cranial nerve monitoring beyond the facial and auditory nerves. *Seminars in Hearing, 14*(2), 163–171.

Barber, H., & Stockwell, C. (1980). *Manual of electronystagmography.* St. Louis: C.V. Mosby Company.

Beck D., & Benecke, J. (1990). Intraoperative facial nerve monitoring: Technical aspects. *Otolaryngology—Head and Neck Surgery, 102,* 270–272.

Boothe, R. Tigges, M., & Wilson, J. (1990). Monkey model of treatment for infantile aphakic amblyopia. *Investigative Ophthalmology and Visual Science, 31*(Suppl.), 279.

Buttner, V., Buttner-Ennever, J. & Henn, V. (1977). Vertical eye movements related to unit activity in rostral mesencephalic reticular formation of the alert monkey. *Brain Research, 130,* 239–252.

Carl, J. (1993). Practical anatomy and physiology of the oculomotor system. In G. Jacobson, C. Newman, & J. Kartush (Eds.), *The handbook of balance function testing* (pp. 53–68). St. Louis: Mosby Year Book Inc.

Carpenter, M. (1985). *Core textbook of neuroanatomy.* Baltimore: Williams and Wilkins.

Dyer, J., & Lee, D. (1984). *Atlas of extraocular muscle surgery.* New York: Praeger Publishers.

Evinger, L., Fuchs, A., & Baker, R. (1977). Bilateral lesions of the medial longitudinal fasciculus in monkeys: Effects of the horizontal and vertical components of voluntary and vestibular induced eye movements. *Experimental Brain Research, 28,* 1-20.

Feldon S., & Burde, R. (1992). The oculomotor system. In W. Hart, Jr. (Ed.), *Adler's physiology of the eye* (pp. 134-183). St. Louis: Mosby Year Book, Inc.

Goldberg, S. (1991). *Ophthalmology made ridiculously simple.* Miami: MedMaster, Inc.

Goldberg, M., Eggers, H., & Gouras, P. (1991). The ocular motor system. In E. Kandel, J. Schwartz, & T. Jessell (Eds.), *Principles of neural science* (pp. 660-678). New York: Elsevier.

Honrubia, V., & Hoffman, L. (1993). Practical anatomy and physiology of the vestibular system. In G. Jacobson, C. Newman, & J. Kartush (Eds.), *The handbook of balance function testing* (pp. 9-52). St. Louis: Mosby Year Book Inc.

Ingram R., Wilson, C., Arnold, P.E., & Dally, S. (1986). Prediction of amblyopia and squint by means of refraction at age 1 year. *British Journal of Ophthalmology, 70,* 12.

Jacobson, G., & Balzer, G. (1992). Basic considerations in intraoperative monitoring. In J. Kartush & K. Bouchard (Eds.), *Neuromonitoring in otology and head and neck surgery* (pp. 21-60). New York: Raven Press, Ltd.

Jacobson, S., Sandberg, M., Effron, M., & Berson, E.L. (1979). Foveal cone electroretinograms in strabismic amblyopia. *Transaction of the Ophthalmological Societies of the United Kingdom, 99,* 353.

Kartush, J., & Bouchard, K. (1992). Intraoperative facial nerve monitoring. In J. Kartush & K. Bouchard (Eds.), *Neuromonitoring in otology and head and neck surgery* (pp. 99-120). New York: Raven Press, Ltd.

Kartush, J. (1989). Electroneurography and intraoperative facial nerve monitoring in contemporary neurotology. *Otolaryngology—Head and Neck Surgery, 101,* 496-503.

Keith R. & Bankaitis, A. (1993). Intraoperative monitoring of the auditory brainstem response and facial nerve. *Current Opinion in Otolaryngology and Head and Neck Surgery, 1*(1), 64-71.

Lenarz, T., & Ernst, A. (1992). Intraoperative monitoring by transtympanic electrocochleography and brainstem electrical response audiometry in acoustic neuroma surgery. *European Archives of Otorhinolaryngology, 249,* 257-262.

Maciewicz, R., & Spencer, R. (1977). Oculomotor and abducens internuclear pathways in the cat. *Developmental Neuroscience, 1,* 99.

Manninen, P., Cuillerier, D., Nantau, D., & Gelb, W. (1992). Monitoring of brainstem functions during vertebral basilar aneurysm surgery. *Anesthesiology, 77,* 681-685.

Martin, J. (1989). *Neuroanatomy text and atlas.* New York: Elsevier Science Publishing Co.

Moller, A. (1992). Intraoperative neurophysiological monitoring. *Neurological Research, 14,* 216-218.

Moller, A., & Moller, B. (1989). Does intraoperative monitoring of auditory evoked potentials reduce incidence of hearing loss as a complication of microvascular decompression of cranial nerves? *Neurosurgery, 24,* 257-263.

Moller, A. (1988). Intraoperative monitoring of cranial motor nerves. In A. Moller (Ed.), *Evoked potentials in intraoperative monitoring* (pp. 99-120). Baltimore: Williams and Wilkins.

Mori, N., Takahashi, H., Yanase, T., & Suzuki, M. (1990). Pressure-supported ventilation for posterior fossa operation. *Journal of Neurosurgery and Anesthesiology, 2,* 28-35.

Nolte, J. (1988). *The human brain.* St. Louis: Mosby Year Book, Inc.

Prass, R. (1992). Intraoperative electromyographic recording. In J. Kartush & K. Bouchard (Eds.) *Neuromonitoring in otology and head and neck surgery* (pp. 81-98). New York: Raven Press, Ltd.

Prass, R., & Luders, H. (1986). Acoustic (loudspeaker) facial electromyographic monitoring: Part 1. *Neurosurgery, 19,* 392-400.

Sacks, J. (1984). The shape of the trochlea. *Archives in Ophthalmology, 102*(69), 933.

Sindou, M., Fobe, J., Ciriano, D., & Fischer, C. (1992). Hearing prognosis and intraoperative guidance of brainstem auditory evoked potential in microvascular decompression. *Laryngoscope, 102,* 678-682.

Wilson-Pauwels, L., Akesson, E., & Stewart, P. (1988). *Cranial nerves: Anatomy and clinical comments.* Toronto: B.C. Decker Inc.

Wolff, E. (1976). *Anatomy of the eye and orbit.* Revised by R. Warwick. Philadelphia: W.B. Saunders Company.

CHAPTER 3

MONITORING THE TRIGEMINAL NERVE

■ AUKSE E. BANKAITIS, M.A. ■
■ ROBERT W. KEITH, Ph.D. ■

Neurosurgical case loads vary significantly from hospital to hospital; yet the objectives and applications of cranial nerve intraoperative monitoring remain universal. Electrophysiologic monitoring of cranial nerves provides surgeons with direct and immediate feedback for the identification and function of pertinent nerves that may inadvertently be damaged from surgical manipulation (Daube & Harper, 1989). The vulnerability of the trigeminal nerve (CN V) during surgical treatment of trigeminal neuralgia in which portions of sensory nerve fibers are deliberately sectioned or in cases of posterior fossa tumors such as large vestibular schwannomas (acoustic neuromas) or meningiomas may be significantly reduced with intraoperative cranial nerve monitoring.

From our own experience, intraoperative monitoring of the trigeminal nerve is accompanied by monitoring of other cranial nerves and typically coincides with various surgical procedures involving removal of masses such as petrous ridge meningiomas, fourth ventricle tumors, large cerebellopontine angle tumors, middle fossa infiltrating meningiomas, as well as brainstem arterial venous malformations (AVM). Although preoperative diagnoses may indicate when to monitor the trigeminal nerve, the integration of such knowledge with the anatomy of CN V is necessary in planning and executing a successful intraoperative protocol.

ANATOMY OF THE TRIGEMINAL NERVE (CN V)

Composed mainly of afferent fibers, the trigeminal nerve is the principle sensory nerve of the head, ultimately transmitting tactile, proprioceptive, along with pain and temperature information from the head to the cerebral cortex, cerebellum, and reticular formation (Matzke & Foltz, 1983; Nolte, 1988).

SENSORY COMPONENTS OF THE TRIGEMINAL NERVE

The primary sensory or afferent fibers of the trigeminal nerve are distributed peripherally via three main branches: the ophthalmic (V1), maxillary (V2), and mandibular (V3) divisions. The areas supplied by these three divisions are very distinct. Generally, each division supplies the upper portion of the face (forehead and cornea), the mid-portion of the face (i.e., nose, cheek, upper lip, and teeth) and the lower portion of the face (jaw, chin, lower lip, and lower teeth), respectively. Once the afferent fibers pierce though the cranium, the fibers enter the lateral portion of the mid pons by penetrating the middle cerebellar peduncle and course toward anatomically and functionally distinct cell bodies of the trigeminal ganglion. From the cell bodies of the trigeminal ganglion, pain and temperature, discriminative touch, and proprioceptive sensations from the face are transmitted to the postcentral gyrus by various trigeminal pathways.

SENSORY DEFICITS RESULTING FROM VARIOUS LESIONS

An occlusion of the posterior inferior cerebellar artery (PICA) often results in a complex set of sensory and motor deficits collectively referred to as lateral medullary syndrome, or Wallenberg's syndrome (Martin, 1989). The sensory deficits characteristic of Wallenberg's syndrome include deficits in pain and temperature senses of the ipsilateral face because the neurons that mediate these senses are located in the lateral medulla (Moller, 1989).

   An aneurysm of the internal carotid artery within the cavernous sinus may irritate the V1 and possibly the V2 branch of the trigeminal nerve resulting in severe pain in the territories supplied by these nerves (Duus, 1989). Characterized by attacks of sharp, agonizing, excruciating pain, trigeminal neuralgia (tic douloureux) is often limited to a territory supplied by one or more branches of the trigeminal nerve (Nolte, 1988). Between attacks, no significant abnormalities can be found. There is frequently a "trigger zone" in the involved area, where tactile stimulation may precipitate an attack (Terrence, 1987). The shooting pain occurs suddenly and with great severity.

Within the cranium, damage to the trigeminal nerve may occur from various conditions, including meningitis, pontocerebellar angle tumors, and various types of otitis (Duus, 1989). Trismus, a tonic spasm of the masticatory muscles, is often a result of either acute encephalitic lesions in the pons, rabies, tetanus, or other conditions. This results in such abnormally intense muscular tension that an individual may not be able to open the mouth (lockjaw).

MOTOR PORTION OF THE TRIGEMINAL NERVE

The trigeminal motor nucleus, the only efferent nucleus associated with the trigeminal nerve, originates within the midlateral tegmentum of the rostral pons. Fibers arising from the trigeminal motor nucleus emerge as a separate motor root and exit from the cranium through the foramen ovale, enter the mandibular branch of the trigeminal nerve, and distribute peripherally with the mandibular division (Nolte, 1988). The nerve branches extensively to innervate muscles of mastication, including the temporalis, masseter, mylohyoid, medial and lateral pterygoids, and the anterior belly of the digastric muscle (Gilman & Winans, 1982; Martin, 1989). Each motor nucleus of the trigeminal nerve receives bilateral influences from the primary motor cortex. This bilateral control results in the tandem coordination of the muscles of mastication on both sides of the mouth during such activities as chewing (Martin, 1989).

MOTOR DEFICITS RESULTING FROM VARIOUS LESIONS

Lesions of the trigeminal nerve most often result in paralysis of the muscles of mastication on the affected side. Peripheral lesions of the nerve result in flaccid paralysis of corresponding chewing muscles, which can be recognized by feeling the size and tautness of the masseter muscles as the jaws are clenched (Gilman & Winans, 1982). Flaccid paralysis is often followed by atrophy of the muscles. If the patient is asked to open the mouth and to push the chin forward, the chin will deviate to the side of the paralysis because of the predominance of the pterygoid muscle of the opposite side (Duus, 1989). Also, the reflex of the masseter muscle will be absent on the paralyzed side.

Unilateral lesions of the motor cortex will not produce any marked deficits, because the motor nucleus of each side receives input from upper motor neurons originating in both the left and the right motor cortex (Martin, 1989). However, an upper motor neuron lesion rostral to the pons may result in an exaggerated jaw jerk reflex (Gilman & Winans, 1982).

INTRAOPERATIVE MONITORING TECHNIQUES

As the trigeminal nerve comprises both motor and sensory fibers, several distinctly different monitoring techniques may be incorporated in the intraoperative monitoring protocol. According to Daube and Harper (1989), monitoring methods can be divided into four categories: compound muscle action potentials (CMAP), compound nerve action potentials (NAP), somatosensory cortical evoked potential (SCEP), and electromyography (EMG).

COMPOUND MUSCLE AND COMPOUND NERVE ACTION POTENTIALS

Monitoring CMAP or NAP with direct stimulation of the exposed CN V can provide relatively rapid information to a surgeon about functional nerve integrity. Monitoring CMAP involves direct stimulation of the motor fibers of the trigeminal nerve with a handheld stimulating probe by the surgeon, with the NAP relying on direct stimulation of the trigeminal nerve sensory fibers. An evoked potential averaging unit, such as the Biologic Brain Atlas, may be used to record both the CMAP and the NAP as long as the response electrodes are located at a muscle innervated by the trigeminal nerve or along the length of the nerve referenced to an electrode on the scalp, respectively (Daube & Harper, 1989).

SOMATOSENSORY CORTICAL EVOKED POTENTIALS

When a cranial or peripheral nerve is electrically stimulated, the action potential propagates along the axons both distally (orthodromic) and proximally (antidromic) (Richmond & Mahla, (1985). As the trigeminal nerve contains motor and sensory fibers, direct stimulation of an intact trigeminal nerve will result in the contraction of the muscle innervated by the nerve. In addition, the sensory fibers of the trigeminal nerve will also respond to direct electrical stimulation by transmitting tactile and pain information to the primary sensory cortex located in the contralateral parietal lobe. As a result, monitoring the sensory aspect of the trigeminal nerve may be accomplished with SCEP.

As with any type of evoked potential monitoring, a signal averaging computer available for monitoring evoked potentials is suitable to monitor trigeminal nerve SCEP. In accordance with the international 10–20 electrode placement system, response electrodes should be placed at FPZ and either C3 or C4, depending on whether the right or the left trigeminal nerve is at-risk. In the absence of established universal parameters, Richmond and Mahla (1985) suggest a 20 ms time window and stimulation rate of 2 per second at an intensity level of 1.0 mA with a stimulus duration of 150 μsec and the filters set at 30–3000 Hz.

ELECTROMYOGRAPHY

EMG is an appropriate technique for monitoring the motor portion of the trigeminal nerve. EMG records the potentials generated by muscle, potentials that occur in response to mechanical or metabolic irritation of the nerve innervating the muscle (Daube & Harper, 1989). Most of the cases we monitor involve on-line monitoring of the auditory brainstem response (ABR), SCEP, and EMG. With cranial nerve monitoring, as EMG techniques do not rely on multiple signal averaging, we prefer to use EMG over CMAP, NAP, and SCEP; however, the combined use of EMG and SCEP for monitoring mixed cranial nerves has been advocated (Jannetta, Moller, & Moller, 1984), especially during acoustic neuroma resection or decompression and vascular decompression of several cranial nerves.

EQUIPMENT

Although a number of devices are available to monitor cranial nerve EMG activity, we use the Nerve Integrity Monitor-2 (NIM-2, Xomed-Treace, Inc., Jacksonville, Florida; Figure 3–1). The NIM-2 directs detected EMG signals

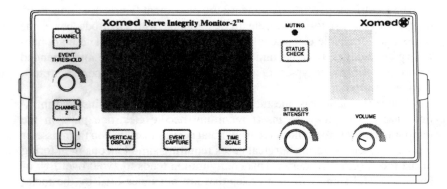

FIGURE 3–1. The Nerve Integrity Monitor-2 (NIM-2, Xomed-Treace, Inc., Jacksonville, Florida) directs detected EMG activity to an oscilloscope that generates a visual representation of muscle activity on a central screen.

to an oscilloscope to generate not only a visual representation of muscle activity, but immediate auditory EMG feedback as well. The audible EMG feature of the NIM-2 allows the most rapid and immediate interpretation of responses within the context of surgical events (Kartush, 1989) by decreasing delays associated with signal averaging. The audibility of the EMG responses also decreases the risk of misunderstandings (Moller, 1989) of spoken exchanges between the intraoperative personnel and surgical staff. In addition, the NIM-2 EMG system is equipped with a muting system that automatically eliminates electrical artifact associated with the extensive use of electrocautery equipment during neurosurgery (Bankaitis & Keith, 1993).

ANESTHESIA

Communication with the anesthesiologist prior to and throughout the surgical procedure is a necessity. Long-acting muscle relaxants or neuromuscular blocking agents must be avoided. During the initial patient preparation and induction of anesthesia, paralyzing drugs may be utilized. However, once the structures to be monitored are surgically approached, paralyzing drug effects must be reversed. Even low doses of muscle relaxants that block nerve responses from direct electrical stimulation may compromise small amplitude EMG responses associated with mechanical manipulation (Kartush & Bouchard, 1992).

ELECTRODES

Although various types of electrodes are available, for intraoperative monitoring of the trigeminal nerves, subdermal needle electrodes are preferred. Needle electrodes permit rapid and secure placement (Kartush & Bouchard, 1992). In contrast to surface electrodes applied with electrode paste, the impedance of needle electrodes does not change over time. These are necessary advantages, because limited patient preparation time and extended recording sessions are typical of most surgical cases that incorporate intraoperative monitoring.

Once the patient is anesthetized, needle electrodes are inserted intramuscularly. We prefer to insert recording needle electrode pairs in the temporalis muscle to monitor the trigeminal nerve rather than in the masseter muscle, especially during surgical cases requiring simultaneous monitoring of the facial (CN VII) nerve. This configuration tends to avoid overflow of far-field EMG signals from muscles that are not innervated by the facial nerve (i.e., masseter). Occasionally, however, certain surgical approaches require an incision and retraction of the temporalis muscle. In this case, monitoring within the vicinity of the temporalis muscle is not possible. In this situation, we use the masseter muscle as the response site for monitoring the trigeminal nerve.

Once electrodes are inserted into the proper response sites, functional electrode integrity must be verified. As with any electrophysiological test, obtaining the lowest possible electrode impedances is desirable (less than 5,000 ohms). Impedances should be balanced resulting in the interelectrode impedances of less than 1,000 ohms. These standards reduce the "antenna-like" quality of electrode input wires as higher impedances are more suscept-ible to the detection of electromagnetic noise (Prass, 1992).

Once normal electrode impedances have been achieved, we further verify electrode function with a "touch" or "tap" test (Beck & Benecke, 1990). Touching or tapping the vicinity of the electrode response area should register an audible and visual response from and on the oscilloscopic display of the NIM-2. This simple procedure confirms proper operation of the rec-ording equipment. For further information regarding stimulating probes and interpretation of responses, please refer to Chapter 2.

CASE STUDY

This is a report of a 63-year-old female with a preoperative diagnosis of a men-ingioma of the petrous ridge. The patient underwent a petrous petrosal cran-iotomy for removal of the tumor. Electrophysiologic monitoring of brainstem function during tumor removal was accomplished through ABR testing, with insert earphones placed in each ear and median nerve SCEP with stimulus electrodes placed near the right and left median nerve at the wrist. Scalp recording electrodes were placed appropriately at A1, A2, C3, and C4 referenced to FZ.

CN IV, V, VI, VII, and XI were also monitored in the following way. A subdermal electrode was placed near the medial rectus and a subdermal elec-trode was placed near the lateral rectus muscles of the eye. The placement was inside the orbital rim of the medial canthus and along the outer rim of the lateral canthus. Reference subdermal electrodes were placed in the opposite forehead. In addition, for monitoring of CN V, response electrodes were placed in the masseter muscle at the angle of the jaw. CN VII was monitored with response electrodes in the orbicularis oris muscle with CN XI monitored with response electrode pairs in the trapezius muscle.

Ongoing monitoring of background EMG activity showed fluctuating levels with the bipolar near CN V and VII. For example, baseline background EMG activity typically remained at 15–19 μV. However, during tumor re-moval background levels characterized by overall increase in EMG activity went to 90 μV and remained there for several minutes. The EMG activity always returned to baseline. CN V was identified by stimulating in the tumor at 0.05 mA at 4 pulses per second, using the Prass monopolar stimulator. The response level was 230 μV. Increase in the background EMG activity occurred with irrigation, but activity always returned to baseline levels. After tumor removal, CN V and VII were stimulated again to ensure their viability. Responses were present to stimulation of both cranial nerves at levels of approximately 250 μV. In addition, all baseline activity had returned to 19 μV. It appeared that CN V and VII were intact and functioning at the time of closure and predicted good postoperative function.

REFERENCES

Bankaitis, A., & Keith, R. (1993). Cranial nerve monitoring beyond the facial and auditory nerves. *Seminars in Hearing, 14*(2), 163–171.

Beck, D., & Benecke, J. (1990). Intraoperative facial nerve monitoring: Technical aspects. *Otolaryngology—Head and Neck Surgery, 102*, 270–272.

Daube, J. R., & Harper, C. M. (1989). Surgical monitoring of cranial and peripheral nerves. In J. E. Desmedt (Ed.), *Neuromonitoring in surgery*. Amsterdam: Elsevier Science Publishers (B.V. Biomedical Division).

Duus, P. (1989). *Topical diagnosis in neurology*. New York: Thieme Medical Publishers, Inc.

Gilman, S., & Winans, S. (1982). *Essentials of clinical neuroanatomy and neurophysiology*. Philadelphia: F.A. Davis Company.

Jannetta, P., Moller A., & Moller., M. (1984). Technique for hearing preservation in small acoustic neuromas. *Annals of Surgery, 200*, 513–523.

Kartush, J., & Bouchard, K. (1992). Intraoperative facial nerve monitoring. In J. Kartush & K. Bouchard (Eds.), *Neuromonitoring in otology and head and neck surgery*. New York: Raven Press, Ltd.

Kartush, J. (1989). Electroneurography and intraoperative facial nerve monitoring in contemporary neurotology. *Otolaryngology Head and Neck Surgery, 101*, 496–503.

Martin, J. (1989). *Neuroanatomy text and atlas*. New York: Elsevier Publishing.

Matzke, H., & Foltz, F. (1983). Trigeminal Pathways. In *Synopsis of neuroanatomy*. New York: Oxford University Press.

Moller, A. (1989). Intraoperative electrophysiological monitoring during microvascular decompression of cranial nerves V, VII, and VIII. In J. E. Desmedt (Ed.), *Neuromonitoring in surgery* (pp. 209–218). New York: Elsevier Science Publishers B.V. (Biomedical Division).

Nolte, J. (1988). *The human brain*. St. Louis: Mosby Year Book, Inc.

Prass, R. (1992). Intraoperative electromyographic recording. In J. Kartush & K. Bouchard (Eds.), *Neuromonitoring in otology and head and neck surgery* (pp. 81–98). New York: Raven Press.

Richmond, I., & Mahla, M. (1985). Use of antidromic recording to monitor facial nerve function intraoperatively. *Neurosurgery, 16*(4), 458–462.

Terrence, C. (1987). Differential diagnosis of trigeminal neuralgia. In G. Fromm (Ed.), *The medical and surgical management of trigeminal neuralgia* (pp. 43–68). New York: Futura Publishing Company.

CHAPTER 4

MONITORING THE FACIAL NERVE

■ IAN WINDMILL, Ph.D. ■
■ KEN HENRY, Ph.D. ■

The primary function of the facial nerve (CN VII) is to provide motor innervation for the muscles of facial expression. The facial nerve also carries general visceral fibers that innervate the lacrimal, submandibular, and sublingual glands.

Interruption or damage to the facial nerve may result in reduced or absent facial movement, loss of sensation near the ears, decreased or absent taste, or decreased or absent tearing or salivary action. Functionally, a complete unilateral facial paralysis makes it difficult to eat or drink. Ocular problems, such as drying of the cornea, may arise from loss of motor function of the eyelids.

In addition to the physical effects, patients may also experience significant psychological trauma due to the perceived disfigurement that accompanies a loss of facial motor function. Injury to the facial nerve, therefore, can have severe and debilitating results.

Intraoperative facial nerve monitoring (IFNM) represents a significant adjunct to otologic and skull base surgery. IFNM is frequently employed during surgical procedures involving the middle and posterior fossa, the temporal bone, the parotid gland, or any procedure that places the facial nerve at risk for iatrogenic injury.

Using IFNM allows trauma or injury to the nerve to be detected in "real time." This can lead to alterations in the surgical procedure or appropriate intervention to prevent permanent loss of facial nerve function. IFNM assists the surgeon by identifying the facial nerve within the surgical field and by differentiating the nerve from surrounding tissue.

IFNM meets the following clinical objectives (Niparko & Kileny, 1988):

1. Assisting in distinguishing the facial nerve from regional cranial nerves and from adjacent soft tissue and tumor.
2. Facilitation of tumor excision by electrically mapping regions of the tumor not containing the facial nerve.
3. Early detection of surgical trauma to the facial nerve with immediate feedback to the surgeon.
4. Confirmation of nerve stimulability at the completion of the procedure to prognosticate facial nerve function.
5. Identification of the site and degree of neural degeneration in selected patients undergoing nerve exploration.

ANATOMY AND PHYSIOLOGY OF THE FACIAL NERVE

The major portion of the facial nerve (CN VII) consists of axons whose cell bodies are located in the facial nerve nucleus in the brainstem and whose terminal endings are located at the muscles of the face. The majority of fibers that make up the facial nerve are motor efferents. A small portion of CN VII carries parasympathetic fibers to the salivary and lacrimal glands. The remainder of the fibers that comprise CN VII are afferent and carry sensory information from the external ear canal and pinnae, as well as taste sensation from the palate and anterior two-thirds of the tongue to the brain. Collectively, the parasympathetic fibers and the sensory afferents are known as the nervous intermedius.

Only the motor component of the facial nerve is monitored during surgical procedures and, therefore, the remainder of this chapter's anatomical descriptions will be limited to the motor pathways. Further descriptions of the sensory portion of the nerve will not be presented, as no procedure currently exists to monitor this aspect of the facial nerve intraoperatively. For an in-depth review of the anatomy and physiology of the facial nerve the reader is referred to May (1986).

INTRACRANIAL FACIAL NERVE ANATOMY

Motor control of facial expression is mediated within the premotor and primary motor cortices. Signals are sent via corticobulbar fibers that travel through the internal capsule to the facial nerve nucleus in the brainstem (Figure 4–1). The facial nerve nucleus is located in the pontine tegmentum of the brainstem and receives input signals from both cortices. Axons leaving the facial nerve nucleus course dorsally, loop around abducens nucleus (CN VI), and exit the brainstem on the ventral aspect at the pontine medullary junction. The facial nerve courses across the subarachnoid space of the posterior cranial fossa together with the auditory and vestibular fibers of the vestibulocochlear nerve (CN VIII). In close proximity to the facial and vestibulocochlear nerves is the anterior inferior cerebellar artery.

The facial and vestibulocochlear nerves and one branch of the anterior inferior cerebellar artery enter the petrous portion of the temporal bone via

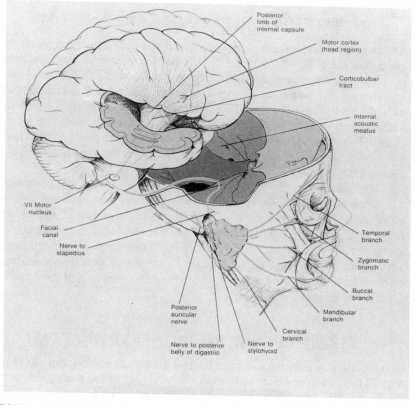

FIGURE 4–1. Motor component of the facial nerve. From *Cranial nerves: Anatomy and clinical comments,* p. 84, by L. Wilson-Pawels, E. T. Akesson, and P. A. Stewart, 1988, Toronto: B. C. Decker. Copyright 1988 by B. C. Decker. Reprinted with permission.

the internal auditory canal (IAC). As the vestibulocochlear nerve enters the IAC, it divides into two identifiable segments, the cochlear nerve and vestibular nerve. The facial nerve generally occupies a superior and anterior position in the IAC. The cochlear nerve fibers sit in an inferior anterior position, with the vestibular nerve fibers residing in a more posterior position. Importantly, one must expect variation in these anticipated locations. Although anatomical descriptions are useful in determining landmarks and relationships, variations are common.

Although the facial nerve is fairly distinguishable within the IAC, the vestibular and cochlear nerves are less well defined. The presence of a mass lesion, such as a vestibular schwannoma (acoustic tumor) within the IAC may further blur the typical anatomical positions and the definition of the nerves.

INTRATEMPORAL FACIAL NERVE ANATOMY

The facial and vestibulocochlear nerves course together for approximately 1 cm within the IAC, after which CN VIII divides to enter the vestibular and cochlear end organs and the CN VII enters the facial canal. The facial nerve turns anteriorly and passes above and between the cochlea and semicircular canals. This section of the facial nerve is referred to as the labyrinthine section and is approximately 3 to 5 mm in length. The geniculate ganglion is located in the labyrinthine segment at the external genu. It is here that the facial nerve gives off a branch known as the greater petrosal nerve, which continues to course anteriorly.

The motor fibers for facial innervation make an abrupt turn posteriorly. The nerve courses past the vestibule of the inner ear and under the semicircular canals. This section of the nerve is known as the tympanic segment and is 10 to 12 mm in length. The facial nerve passes medial to the middle ear space just above the footplate of the stapes. At this point the nerve takes an abrupt turn inferiorly for approximately 12 to 14 mm through the mastoid, referred to as the vertical segment. It is within this section that the stapedial branch and chorda tympani arise.

EXTRATEMPORAL FACIAL NERVE ANATOMY

The facial nerve exits the temporal bone at the stylomastoid foramen (SMF). The SMF is located posterior to the inferior aspect of the pinna. The nerve courses slightly laterally and then anteriorly, passing under the lower border of the pinna, over the mandibular ramus and through the parotid gland. Where the facial nerve is intimately involved with the parotid gland, it begins to divide into its many branches.

Five primary branches are typically identified, although the specific patterns and branches vary across individuals (Figure 4-1). In general the temporal branch of the facial nerve innervates the frontalis muscle of the forehead. The zygomatic branch innervates the muscles responsible for eye closure, the orbicularis oculi. The buccal branch of the facial nerve innervates the buccinator and, along with the mandibular branch, also innervates the orbicularis oris muscles. The platysma is innervated by the cervical branch of the nerve (May, 1986).

OVERVIEW OF IFNM PROCESS

It is important to follow a logical, step-by-step approach to intraoperative monitoring (Table 4-1). The first step is consultation with the surgeon, the anesthesiologist, and the operating room nursing staff. The type of surgery, the risk to the facial nerve, and related concerns, such as use of auditory feedback, should be discussed with the surgeon. The anesthetic regime and its effect on the intraoperative monitoring should be discussed with the anesthesiologist. The nursing staff should be consulted to discuss placement of equipment, sterilization, and electrical requirements.

It is best to place the monitoring equipment away from all other electrical equipment to avoid unwanted electrical "noise." However, when possible, it is beneficial to place the equipment near the surgeon to facilitate communication between the audiologist and the physician and to allow the surgeon to see the recordings, if desired.

All equipment and supplies should be set up and waiting before the patient enters the operating room. Once the patient is intubated and in position, recording electrodes are placed (see Recording Montage section) and secured. The recording electrodes and EMG system should be immediately verified, using the tap test (Beck & Benecke, 1990). Tapping on the skin immediately above the electrodes should result in artifactual responses displayed on the electromyographic (EMG) system (or a "popping" sound should be heard if auditory feedback is being utilized). Electrode impedance should be checked, with all values less than 5000 ohms and less than 1000 ohms difference between electrodes. Once the tap test and impedances are verified, the nurse is notified and scrubbing, sterilization, and further surgical preparation can continue.

During the surgery, particularly when the risk of facial nerve injury is high, attention to the EMG results is critically important. EMG activity and auditory feedback are analyzed and discussed with the surgeon and correlated with surgical events. Communication should be direct and efficient. Intraoperative events should be correlated with postoperative outcomes.

TABLE 4-1. STEPS IN IFNM PROCESS.

I. Preoperative Planning Stage

    A. Consultation with surgeon
        1. Evaluate indication for IFNM
        2. Review surgical procedure
        3. Select IFNM protocol

    B. Consultation with anesthesiologist
        1. Discuss monitoring objectives
        2. Discuss anesthetic protocol

    C. Consultation with operating room nursing staff
        1. Review goal of IFNM
        2. Discuss equipment or supply needs
        3. Plan equipment setup

II. Operative Stage

    A. Prepare equipment—prior to patient arrival
        1. Set up and test equipment
        2. Prepare electrodes and cables
        3. Prepare supplies—skin cleaner, gloves, tape, and so on.

    B. Prepare patient—after anesthesia and intubation
        1. Clean electrode sites
        2. Attach and anchor sterile electrodes
        3. Position electrode cables away from surgical field
        4. Attach electrodes to monitoring equipment
        5. Test electrode contact, including impedance and tap test

    C. Monitoring process
        1. Optimize stimulation and recording setup (according to protocol)
        2. Establish baseline
        3. Provide feedback to surgeon
        4. Maintain log for postsurgical review

    D. Post surgery
        1. Remove electrodes (with caution)
        2. Remove equipment from O.R.
        3. Compare surgical events with postoperative outcome

CLINICAL APPLICATIONS OF IFNM

INDICATIONS

Surgical procedures for which IFNM can be utilized fall into three categories that generally correspond to the segments of the facial nerve described earlier (Table 4-2). Skull base procedures, such as removal of cerebellar pontine angle tumors, place the intracranial section of the nerve at risk. Temporal bone procedures, such as mastoidectomies (Pensak, Willging, & Keith, 1994) or cochlear implantation, involve risk to the intratemporal aspect of the nerve. Procedures such as parotidectomies pose an injury risk to the extratemporal portion of the nerve.

Skull base procedures may place at risk the segment of the facial nerve from the brainstem through the subarachnoid space up to and including the internal auditory canal. The most common skull base procedures that require IFNM are removal of a cerebellar pontine angle tumor, such as a vestibular schwannoma (acoustic tumor). In these cases, the tumor is located either adjacent to the brainstem or within the IAC and frequently is intimately involved with the facial nerve. IFNM can be utilized by the surgeon to discriminate tumor from facial nerve.

Other surgical procedures of the posterior fossa in which IFNM may play an important role include vascular loop decompression and vestibular nerve section. These procedures often involve direct manipulation of the facial nerve. IFNM may also be useful during trigeminal nerve decompression, in which traction or manipulation of the brainstem or cerebellum may occur. During retraction of the cerebellum, the intracranial segment of the facial nerve may be injured from stretching.

The facial nerve is at risk for iatrogenic injury during surgery of the temporal bone, as the exact location of the nerve cannot always be appreciated during the operative procedure. Although the general course of the nerve is similar across individuals, the exact course does vary. Landmarks that help distinguish the facial nerve canal are also variable, particularly in children where the landmarks may not be fully developed or discernable. Monitoring aids the surgeon by providing an early warning system when the facial nerve becomes unexpectedly exposed within the surgical field.

For example, a facial nerve recess approach, entering the middle ear through the mastoid, is used for cochlear implantation. During drilling of the mastoid, the facial nerve is identified and avoided. IFNM allows the surgeon to determine the location of the facial nerve and make appropriate judgments regarding the operative approach that will avoid injury to the nerve.

Another example of temporal bone surgery in which IFNM can be employed is facial nerve decompression (Gantz, Gmur, & Fisch, 1982). This

TABLE 4–2. INDICATIONS FOR IFNM.

I. Intracranial
   A. Cerebellopontine angle tumor
   B. Vestibular schwannoma (acoustic tumor)
   C. Microvascular decompression
   D. Trigeminal nerve resection
   E. Vestibular nerve section

II. Intratemporal
   A. Facial nerve decompression
   B. Mastoidectomy
   C. Tympanoplasty
   D. Cochlear implantation
   E. Translabyrnthine approach to posterior fossa
   F. Labyrinthectomy

III. Extratemporal
   A. Parotidectomy
   B. Head and neck dissection
   C. Congenital aural atresia

procedure is designed to relieve pressure on a nerve segment within the temporal bone. By exposing various segments of the nerve, systematic mapping of nerve responses can pinpoint the portion of the facial nerve to be decompressed. Other surgeries of the temporal bone for which IFNM can be employed include mastoidectomies, labyrinthectomies, and translabyrnthine approaches to the posterior fossa.

The third major category for IFNM application is surgeries involving the extratemporal portion of the facial nerve. The most common operative procedure in this area is the parotidectomy (Schwartz & Rosenberg, 1992). In most individuals, the facial nerve passes through or begins to branch within the body of the parotid gland. After exposing the gland, the surgeon can use IFNM to distinguish the nerve from adjacent tissue and can map the course of the branches of the nerve. By stimulating segments of the nerve trunk or branches and by monitoring the EMG response, iatrogenic injury can be avoided.

ANESTHETIC EFFECTS

An important factor that must be considered during IFNM is the use of anesthetic agents that induce muscle paralysis. As IFNM records responses from the muscles of the face, any induced paralysis will abolish or attenuate the electromyographic response. Consultation with the anesthesiologist is critically important before initiating IFNM.

Three types of anesthetic agents may be used during a surgical procedure: those that produce amnesia (unconsciousness), those that produce analgesia (insensitivity to pain), and those that depress neuromuscular transmission or depress muscle tone (muscle relaxation or paralysis) (Schwartz, Bloom, Pratt, & Costello, 1988). Of the three, those that result in muscle relaxation or induced paralysis are of most concern during IFNM. Obviously, the use of agents that suppress motor activity will have a profound effect on the ability to record facial electromyographic activity. Neuromuscular blockers interrupt the transmission link between the terminal ending of nerves and motor end plates of muscles. Essentially, these drugs block the ability of neurotransmitter to produce depolarization in the muscle, either through constant depolarization of the postsynaptic receptors or by directly blocking the postsynaptic receptors. In either case, the net effect is loss of ability of the muscles to react to neural signals (Hogan, 1992).

Before any IFNM procedure, the anesthesiologist should be informed as to the intention of using IFNM, so that an appropriate anesthetic course can be planned. Often, a short-acting neuromuscular blocking agent is used at the beginning of surgery to facilitate intubation by relaxing the muscles of the larynx and trachea. Fortunately, these agents will be entirely dissipated by the time the facial nerve is exposed. (For a complete discussion of anesthesia considerations, please see Chapter 13, Anesthesia and Intraoperative Monitoring.)

INTRAOPERATIVE METHODS

IFNM is most often accomplished by detecting the electromyographic activity (electrical activity associated with muscle movement) of facial muscles that occurs with stimulation of the facial nerve. IFNM is achieved by recording the activity directly from the facial muscles innervated by the VIIth nerve rather than the motor unit action potentials from the nerve itself.

The specific protocol employed for IFNM is dependent on the type of surgery, the surgical site, and the risk of injury to the facial nerve. Two types of IFNM are commonly employed.

The first type involves continuously monitoring the bioelectric baseline activity of the facial musculature. Injury, direct mechanical manipulation of the nerve, changes in temperature or traction on the nerve all result in fluctuations in electrical responses (compound muscle action potentials) from the facial muscles.

The responses are characterized by a variety of patterns that can be visually observed on an oscillographic monitor, routed to a loudspeaker to provide auditory feedback, or both (Prass & Luders, 1986). The responses have been characterized as "bursts," or "trains," and have distinct oscillographic patterns and auditory sounds. These responses can then be correlated with events within the surgical field.

The second commonly employed method for IFNM uses a stimulus/response paradigm whereby an electrical simulator is used to induce a motor response in the facial musculature. Hand held probe units with specific electrical output characteristics can be used to "search and map" the surgical field. Contact between the stimulating probe and the facial nerve will elicit facial movements, which are recorded and displayed. The recorded response is in the form of a compound action potential (CAP). This method is used when the surgeon needs to differentiate the facial nerve from surrounding tissue (Kartush, Niparko, Bledsoe, Graham, & Kemink, 1985).

As previously stated, the decision as to which type of monitoring procedure to use is dictated by the type of procedure, the surgical site, and the risk of injury to the nerve. If the surgery involves an otherwise healthy, likely uninvolved nerve with minimal risk for injury, the nonstimulating form of IFNM may be chosen. For example, cochlear implantation utilizes an approach in which the surgeon drills through the temporal bone, identifies the facial nerve, and enters the middle ear space. Typically, there is minimal risk of facial nerve injury during cochlear implantation. Baseline electrical activity can be monitored for responses that would signal temperature changes (from drilling) or mechanical contact with the nerve as the surgeon approaches, identifies, and manages the facial nerve. The surgeon may employ the stimulate/response paradigm by periodically halting the drilling and electrically stimulating tissue to see if the facial nerve is present within the surgical site.

Both types of monitoring are typically used within the same surgical procedure. Alternating monitoring procedures during surgery is manageable, and the audiologist should be prepared to employ both protocols. Protocols can be developed based on the type of surgery, the surgical site, and the degree of risk of injury to the nerve. Table 4–3 lists recommendations for establishing a protocol. However, a final protocol should consider site-specific factors and personal preferences.

RECORDING TECHNIQUE

RECORDING ELECTRODES

Facial nerve EMG potentials can be recorded by utilizing surface electrodes or needle electrodes (Figure 4–2). Surface electrodes, like those employed for

TABLE 4-3. RECOMMENDED STIMULATION AND RECORDING PARAMETERS FOR INTRAOPERATIVE FACIAL NERVE MONITORING.

Recording Parameters		Stimulation Parameters	
Parameter	**Recommended**	**Parameter**	**Recommended**
Electrode type	Teflon-coated EMG needle	Stimulus	Rectangular pulse
Electrode montage		Current	Constant
Channel one	Paired at obicularis oris		
Channel two	Paired at obicularis oculi	Stimulus duration	100 μsec
Ground	High forehead (Fpz)		
Reference	High forehead (Fpz)	Rate	2 to 10/sec
Gain	10,000	Intensity	0.2 to 2mA
High cut filter	500 to 3000 Hz	Type	
		General	Monopolar
Low cut filter	5 to 100 Hz	Specific	Bipolar
Sweep			
With stimulation	20 to 100 msec		
Without stimulation	500 to 1000 msec		
Artifact rejection	Off		
Audio feedback	On		

auditory brainstem response (ABR) testing or electroencephalographic (EEG) recording have a relatively large surface area that yields a lower current impedance. Although these electrodes are useful in detecting large amplitude synchronous EMG activity, the EMG responses obtained can be from a broad, nonspecific surface areas and therefore result in erroneous interpretations. In addition, it can be difficult to maintain the electrodes directly on the skin surface. Surface electrodes require paste or gel as an impedance medium between the skin and the electrode. Electrode gels increase the risk of the electrode becoming dislodged because of gel viscosity. Electrode paste has a tendency to dry over time and, therefore, may not remain viable during a lengthy procedure.

Subdermal needle electrodes are preferred over surface electrodes for recording EMG activity during IFNM. Subdermal needle electrodes are often chosen as they provide low impedance and are easy to use. Needle electrodes are quick to insert. They can be gas or steam sterilized and are somewhat

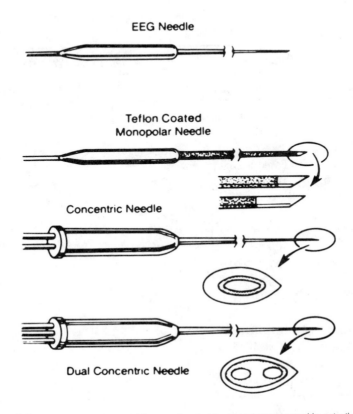

FIGURE 4–2. Needle electrodes used in recording facial nerve electromyographic potentials. From *Neuromonitoring in Otology and Head and Neck Surgery,* p. 88, by J. Kartush and K. Bouchard, 1992, New York: Raven Press. Copyright 1992 by Raven Press, Ltd. Reprinted with permission.

reusable. However, when subdermal needle electrodes are used, one may record unwanted bioelectrical activity from the masseter muscle (which is innervated by the trigeminal nerve).

"Hook wire" electrodes (Figure 4–3) can be used for facial nerve monitoring as well as monitoring motor function associated with other cranial nerves (Prass, 1992). These electrodes are made from a fine gauge medical wire with a Teflon coating. A small area of the terminal end is stripped of insulation and folded to form a "hook." Using a hypodermic needle, the electrodes are inserted into tissue (Beck, 1993). The "hook" prevents the needles from becoming accidently dislodged during the surgical procedure.

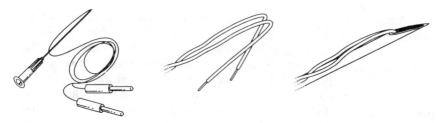

FIGURE 4–3. Bipolar hook wire electrodes for recording EMG potentials. From "Facial Nerve Electrophysiology: Electroneurography and Facial Nerve Monitoring" by D. L. Beck, 1993, *Seminars in Hearing, 14*, p. 129. Copyright 1993 by Thieme Medical Publishers. Reprinted with permission.

Teflon-coated EMG needles used in diagnostic EMG examinations can also be used for monitoring. The shaft of the needle is insulated up to the terminus of the needle. The insulated shaft minimizes surface contact with the skin or subcutaneous tissue. Artifacts from skin potentials are minimized and the specificity of the receptor field is greatly improved.

Of the various types of electrodes available for IFNM, Teflon-coated subdermal needles are the most popular for recording evoked EMG activity intraoperatively. Although not as stable as hook wire electrodes, subdermal needle electrodes do provide greater stability than surface electrodes. Subdermal needles are easier to remove than hooked electrodes at the completion of the surgery. All electrodes utilized for IFNM should be sterile prior to use. Disposable electrodes are recommended to maximize patient protection.

The use of needle electrodes (either subdermal needle or bipolar hook-wire) increases the risk of exposure of the clinician to blood-borne pathogens. Gloves should be worn to insert and remove the electrodes. Caution is advised in handling electrodes. Disposable electrodes should be considered, as the likelihood of an accidental needle stick is decreased because of immediate disposal. Employing reusable needle electrodes requires cleaning and resterilization techniques, both requiring additional handling of the needles. Disposable electrodes also eliminate the opportunity for patient-to-patient contamination.

RECORDING MONTAGE

Monopolar and bipolar electrode montage refers to the recording array, or the inputs to the equipment, used in facial nerve monitoring or other electrophysiologic procedures. The electrode connections to the inverting and noninverting inputs, also known as active and reference inputs, to a differential amplifier are known as a montage (French: to mount).

A bipolar recording montage utilizes paired inputs to record electrophysiologic activity from the same electrical generator. In the case of IFNM, a bipolar montage would use inputs from a pair of electrodes inserted in the same facial muscle. A bipolar montage is advantageous because the recorded activity is site-specific. There is almost no risk of myogenic artifact from the muscles of mastication or from skin potentials. However, interaction of the potentials recorded from each electrode may theoretically result in a distorted waveform, or a "cancellation effect," in which no waveform is discernable.

A monopolar montage is a recording arrangement in which only one of the electrodes is placed in or on the site of interest. The second electrode is located in "electrically silent" tissue away from the site of interest. Waveforms recorded using a monopolar montage may be contaminated with other bioelectrical potentials.

The choice of recording montage depends on the surgical procedure, the type of equipment in use (single versus dual channel), and the objective of the monitoring. A conventional montage, particularly with equipment that allows recording of two separate events (dual channel), is to record potentials from two facial muscles innervated by different branches of the facial nerve. Typically, the orbicularis oculi, innervated by the zygomatic branch, and the orbicularis oris, innervated by the buccal branch, are chosen for this purpose. An electrode montage in which one recording electrode is placed in the orbicularis oculi muscle and a second electrode in orbicularis oris muscle, with both referenced to an electrode at an inactive site (e.g. high forehead—Fpz) is common.

Another common arrangement for a two-channel montage is placement of a pair of needle electrodes in the orbicularis oculi muscle and the placement of a second pair of electrodes in the orbicularis oris muscles. A pair of electrodes, reference and ground, are placed in the high forehead (Fpz). For equipment that only allows single-channel recording, Moeller and Janetta (1984) recommend recording differentially from the mentalis/orbicularis oris muscle groups of the lower face and the orbicularis oculi/superior frontalis muscle groups of the upper face. By recording from both muscle groups, it is possible to obtain activity from the major branches of the VIIth nerve using a single-channel differential amplifier.

The recommended procedure for electrode positioning and recording includes placement of a pair of Teflon-coated electrodes in both the orbicularis oris (superior to the lip and lateral to the nares) and orbicularis oculi (above the eyebrow) muscle groups (Figure 4–4). A ground and reference pair of electrodes should be placed high on the forehead (Fpz).

After inserting the electrodes, using caution to ensure that no electrodes are in direct contact with each other, they should be taped in place and draped to avoid the surgical field. After the surgical field is sterilized, the electrodes

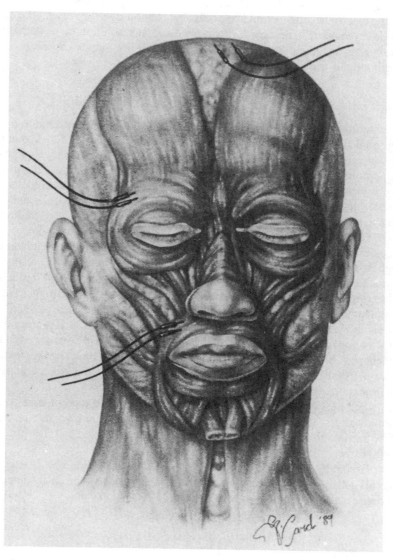

FIGURE 4–4. Position of electrodes for IFNM. Pairs of subdermal electrodes are placed in the obicularis oris and orbicularis oculi muscles. Reference and ground electrodes are placed high in the forehead at the midline in an "electrically neutral" position. From "Electroneurography and Intraoperative Facial Monitoring in Contemporary Neurotology" by J. M. Kartush, 1989, *Otolaryngology Head and Neck Surgery, 101*, p. 501. Copyright 1989 by the American Academy of Otolaryngology—Head and Neck Surgery Foundation, Inc. Reprinted with permission.

will not be accessible for the remainder of the surgery. However, the jack ends of the electrode cables should be accessible. This allows for varying the electrode montage if necessary for improved signal resolution or to manage a broken or dislodged electrode. Electrode extension cables can be used to facilitate this arrangement.

AMPLIFICATION AND FILTER SETTINGS

The neuroelectric signals collected by the electrodes are connected to a differential amplifier, which serves to cancel any similar signals detected at the two electrodes and amplifies only the voltage differences. This is also known as "common mode rejection," in that signals common at the two electrodes are rejected in favor of signals that are different. Although the bioelectric signals generated by muscles are relatively large compared to other neuroelectric signals, a gain of approximately 10,000 must be utilized to make the signal sufficiently large for processing by the monitoring equipment.

The signal passed by the amplifiers must be filtered to remove unwanted signals that may interfere in qualifying or quantifying the EMG response. Typically, EMG responses are low frequency and therefore the low frequency filter (high pass) should be set between 1 and 30 Hz. By using a higher cutoff frequency, the waveform pattern will become slightly distorted, yet will still filter out spurious low frequency artifact such as DC line noise. If preservation of waveform pattern is critical, the frequency filter should be lowered to the extent possible. High frequency filters (low pass) should be set between 1500 Hz and 3000 Hz, although lower frequency settings may be utilized without significant degradation of the signal.

The time base setting will vary depending on the type of monitoring employed. If a stimulator is used, a time base of 20 to 100 msec can be used. If no stimulation is used, the sweep factor can be adjusted to rates of up to 1000 msec.

Generally, no signal averaging is used during IFNM. The bioelectric signals generated by muscles are of sufficient amplitude to be easily detected and discerned within background activity.

STIMULATION TECHNIQUE

As previously noted, two types of monitoring techniques are commonly employed for IFNM. The first involves continuously monitoring the baseline electrical activity for the presence of electromyographic potentials that result without direct, intentional electrical stimulation. The second form of IFNM requires the use of an electrical simulator to elicit a response from the nerve and muscle.

Considerable discussion has been given to the best method for providing direct electrical stimulation for facial nerve mapping or identification (Kartush et al., 1985; Prass & Luders, 1985). Two interactive variables have been identified in these discussions: constant voltage versus constant current and monopolar versus bipolar stimulation.

Effective stimulation of the facial nerve during tumor removal requires that the stimulus be delivered at the same amount of current through either tissue, tumor, or nerve. However, current can be "shunted," or drawn off, by cerebrospinal fluid (CSF), thereby reducing the effective stimulation. Moeller and Janetta (1984) recommend the use of a "constant voltage" stimulator, which maintains the stimulation level even in the presence of shunting. Current levels increase as shunting increases and vice versa. Conversely, Prass and Luders (1985) recommend the use of constant current stimulation with flush tip probes to minimize shunting. Regardless of which method is chosen, either is effective in identifying and stimulating the facial nerve, if used properly. It is probable that specific situations may require different stimulation methods and the indications for each should be developed over time.

Stimulators used to evoke facial nerve activity are either monopolar or bipolar. Monopolar stimulation requires the use of a probe with a single tip and a separate anode electrode. In general, an insulated monopolar stimulator, such as a Prass flush tip probe (Xomed Treace, Jacksonville, Fla.), is preferred to map the general vicinity of the nerve within a given surgical site. In monopolar stimulation, the stimulus current flows between the tip of the stimulator (cathode) to a distally placed anode electrode. If the facial nerve is located between the cathode and anode and the stimulation intensity is sufficient, then depolarization occurs resulting in movement of the facial musculature and a recordable EMG response. However, it is possible that tumor or other tissue being touched by the probe could be falsely identified as nerve, if a response is noted.

Bipolar probes have both the anode and cathode within a single probe tip, and, therefore, the distance between the two points is less than a millimeter. Bipolar stimulation is preferred if selective identification of tissue is necessary. Bipolar probes are often utilized during tissue debulking and differentiation of tissue from nerve, particularly when tumor is being separated from the nerve. Bipolar stimulation reduces the chance of getting a response when not in direct contact with the nerve (false positive error) (Kartush & Bouchard, 1992).

The electrical stimulus used for eliciting a facial nerve response is a rectangular pulse of 100 μsec duration delivered at rates varying between 2 and 5 pulses per second. The intensity of the electrical stimulus varies depending on the proximity of the probe to the facial nerve, but generally varies between 0.05 mA and 2 mA. Rarely is greater than 2 mA required for IFNM. According to Prass (1992), brief pulsed stimulations up to 2 mA using a monopolar stimulator are unlikely to result in neural injury. Initially, a low stimulus intensity (0.4 mA) should be used with current increased systematically as necessary, particularly if intervening tissue is present between the probe and the facial nerve. However, for direct stimulation of the nerve, stimulus intensities should be lowered to levels of 0.1 mA or less.

Inadvertent stimulation of the trigeminal nerve can occur with intracranial stimulation. EMG activity associated with this stimulation can be mistaken for facial nerve activation. Fortunately, intracranial electrical stimulation of the motor portion of the trigeminal nerve results in a quantifiably different response than that arising from stimulation of the facial nerve. The response latency is generally less than 2 msec following intracranial stimulation of the trigeminal nerve, with intracranial stimulation of the facial nerve resulting in a response latency of approximately 5 to 7 msec.

RESPONSE AND INTERPRETATION

In addition to actively stimulating CN VII with electrical impulses, EMG activity arising intraoperatively may be the result of mechanical, thermal, or anesthetic stimulation.

MECHANICAL EVOKED FACIAL EMG ACTIVITY

Mechanical evoked EMG activity is the result of surgical manipulation on or near CN VII. When the nerve is touched, compressed, or stretched, the increase in neural activity produces motor activity that can be recorded from the facial muscles. Activity may also be elicited by surgical devices employed for such activities as electrocautery, laser use, irrigation, or drilling.

Mechanical stimulation produces two distinct patterns of facial nerve EMG activity: trains and bursts (Prass & Luders, 1986). The most common pattern observed intraoperatively with monitoring devices is burst activity (Figure 4–5). This activity is visually represented as a single polyphasic burst of EMG activity and is most often associated with direct manipulation or traction of the nerve. When monitoring includes the use of audio feedback, single "pops" are heard. Burst activity may be seen when cold or warm irrigation is employed on or near the facial nerve. Slow deliberate traction on the nerve is less likely to generate burst activity. Rarely do burst potentials indicate neural insult. Eliciting a burst potential following complete dissection of tumor generally indicates excellent postoperative facial nerve function (Kartush & Bouchard, 1992; Prass & Luders, 1986).

Train potentials are repetitive asynchronous EMG responses (a "corn popping" sound with audio monitoring) frequently associated with medial

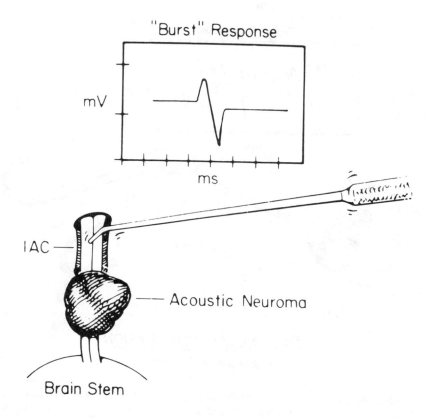

"Burst" Response

mV

ms

IAC

Acoustic Neuroma

Brain Stem

MECHANICAL STIMULATION
Direct Contact

FIGURE 4–5. Burst type response that occurs with direct manipulation of the facial nerve. From "Electroneurography and Intraoperative Facial Monitoring in Contemporary Neurotology" by J. M. Kartush, 1989, *Otolaryngology Head and Neck Surgery, 101,* p. 499. Copyright 1989 by the American Academy of Otolaryngology—Head and Neck Surgery Foundation, Inc. Reprinted with permission.

traction or pressure to the facial nerve (Figure 4–6). Repetitive firing of facial nerve fibers may also occur without any apparent provocation. Although there is no latency between mechanical manipulation and burst activity, there may be a temporal delay between provocation and the onset of a repetitive train. This delay may be as long as minutes (Prass, 1992) after the provocation, which can make identification of an initiating event difficult.

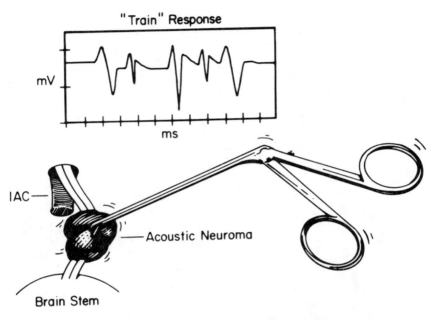

MECHANICAL STIMULATION
Pressure or Traction

FIGURE 4–6. Asynchronous train response that occurs with medial traction or pressure on the facial nerve. From "Electroneurography and Intraoperative Facial Monitoring in Contemporary Neurotology" by J. M. Kartush, 1989, *Otolaryngology Head and Neck Surgery, 101,* p. 500. Copyright 1989 by the American Academy of Otolaryngology—Head and Neck Surgery Foundation, Inc. Reprinted with permission.

Sustained train potentials are thought to indicate some degree of neural insult. These events have been referred to as injury potentials; however, the exact relationship between the activity and injury discharges is not known. Such an association has yet to be confirmed. It is clear, however, that train potentials (repetitive evoked EMG activity) are less useful than burst potentials (nonrepetitive evoked EMG activity) in providing useful information to the surgeon regarding the status of the facial nerve.

THERMALLY EVOKED EMG ACTIVITY

Train potentials may also be evoked by sudden changes in temperature on or about the facial nerve (Kartush & Bouchard, 1992). Electrocautery or laser surgery can heat the nerve. Irrigation with saline can cause sudden cooling. Both can result in the appearance of train potentials. The more sudden the thermal change, the shorter the response latency. Therefore, gradual changes in temperature may be more difficult to correlate with surgical events. Nonetheless, as the facial nerve tissue returns to a normal temperature the train activity subsides.

ELECTRICALLY EVOKED EMG ACTIVITY

Electrical stimulation of the facial nerve and adjacent structures is used for the identification and mapping of the facial nerve and assessment of neural integrity during and after tumor debulking. Adequate electrical stimulation should result in a single polyphasic compound muscle action potential that is precisely timed to the delivery of the electrical stimulus (Figure 4–7). Intracranially, electrical stimulation should result in a large amplitude EMG response having a latency of 5 to 7 msec. However, the latency varies depending on the specific stimulation site. The response latency decreases for direct stimulation within the intratemporal portion of the nerve and is on the order of 2 to 3 msec for stimulation of the extratemporal segment. The response

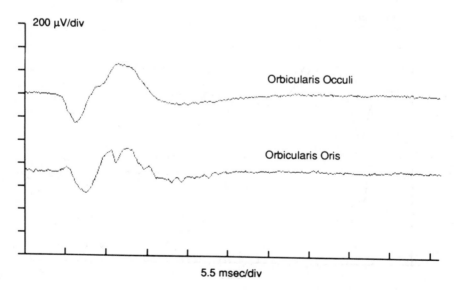

FIGURE 4–7. Typical compound muscle action potentials that result from direct intracranial stimulation of the facial nerve.

amplitude is considerably larger than the EMG potentials resulting from mechanical, thermal, or caloric stimulation. The amplitude of the electrically evoked EMG activity will be dependent on the preoperative status of the nerve (level of nerve excitability), the electrode montage, and the method and intensity of electrical stimulation. In addition, constant stimulation may result in neural fatigue, which will also influence the characteristics of the evoked response.

Figure 4–8 shows normal EMG responses recorded intracranially with bipolar EEG subdermal electrodes from both the orbicularis oculi and orbicularis oris muscles. A 0.4 mA constant current stimulus was applied using a bipolar stimulus probe fashioned after Jacobson and Tew (1987). Response amplitudes exceeded 700 μV. In this case, electrical stimulation helped to identify the facial nerve from surrounding tumor capsule during removal of acoustic neuroma.

Beck, Atkins, Benecke, and Brackmann (1991) show that electrically evoked EMG potentials can be used as a prognostic indicator at the close of surgery. Twenty-eight of 29 patients undergoing acoustic neuroma removal had normal facial motion immediately postoperatively. In addition to having less than 500 μV of ongoing EMG activity, these patients all had EMG

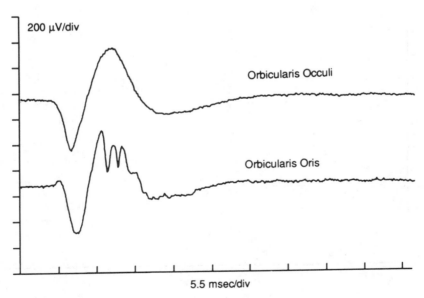

FIGURE 4-8. Compound muscle action potentials from intracranial stimulation using a 0.4 mA constant current. Response latency was 5.0 msec and amplitudes exceeded 700 μV.

contractions greater than 500 μV to a 0.05 mA stimulus at the brainstem at the conclusion of tumor removal.

Electrically evoked EMG responses are analyzed primarily for morphological or amplitude differences. These differences can be between a baseline response and recent stimulation, differences between stimulation in two separate sites, or differences in sequential recordings. For example, distal and proximal responses during removal of an acoustic neuroma can be compared, both to determine if changes in neuron function are occurring or as a post-surgical prognostic indicator. Changes in proximal responses without changes in the distally evoked waveform indicate a change in nerve conduction efficacy. A complete absence of proximal response may signal significant neural injury. In all cases, technical factors such as equipment malfunction or loose electrodes should be ruled out. When used with intratemporal surgical procedures such as facial nerve decompression, electrically evoked responses can be used to identify the site of neural conduction block. As various segments of the nerve are stimulated, obvious amplitude and morphological differences will identify the area of blockage. In addition to amplitude and morphological differences, latency changes should also be apparent in these cases.

CASE EXAMPLE

A 6-year-old child with profound deafness was scheduled to undergo cochlear implantation in the right ear via a facial nerve recess approach. As the temporal bone is not fully mature at this age, identifying landmarks, including the course of the facial nerve, are less distinguishable than for adults. IFNM was planned to assist the otologic surgeon in identifying the facial nerve in its intratemporal course.

A Cadwell 8400 (Cadwell Laboratories, Kennewick, Wa.) evoked potential instrument using an EMG stimulation and recording software program was employed to conduct the monitoring. After intubation, the skin over the electrode sites was cleaned with alcohol. Two sterilized, disposable, Teflon-coated subdermal needle electrodes were placed in the orbicularis oris just superior to the lip on the right side. Two additional subdermal electrodes were placed in the orbicularis oculi at the superior edge of the right eyebrow. A reference electrode was placed on the midline of the forehead just below the hairline. All electrodes were securely taped in place and the jack end of the cables draped over the edge of the operating table. One of each of the electrodes in the orbicularis oris and orbicularis oculi was referenced to the electrode on the forehead (monopolar montage). The remaining electrodes in the orbicularis oculi and oris muscles were used as backups in case of failure of either of the primary electrodes. The electrode from the orbicularis oris muscle was connected to Channel One, with Channel Two receiving input from the orbicularis oris muscle. Impedance was less than 5000 ohms for all electrodes and contact was confirmed by gently tapping on the skin surface directly over the electrodes.

A commercially available, flush tip monopolar stimulator, referenced to an anode electrode, placed at the periphery of the surgical site, was used for stimulation within the surgical field. Constant current stimulation was employed and stimulation parameters were set to 4 pulses per second at an intensity of 0.20 mA.

The EMG instrumentation was set up in the operating room in a location away from potential sources of electrical interference, such as the anesthesia cart. A peripheral video display monitor was provided to allow the surgeon to view the oscillographic recordings, if desired. Acoustical monitoring was also employed. The audiologist provided feedback regarding correlations between acoustic events and the visual display.

During the initial portions of the surgery, the acoustic feedback was turned off because of substantial interference caused by electrocautery. After removal of the skin, muscle, and fascia covering the mastoid area, and at the initiation of drilling into the temporal bone, the acoustic feedback circuit was reinstituted. As the surgery progressed to the point where the risk of injury to the facial became critical, the surgeon would stop drilling and use the stimulator to "explore" the surgical site in an attempt to identify the nerve. If no response was noted, then drilling proceeded. Vague landmarks suggesting the proximity of the facial nerve canal were confirmed by stimulation of the nerve. Having identified the location and course of the nerve, the surgery proceeded without incident and implantation was successful. Baseline electrical activity continued to be monitored for the presence of EMG responses that would suggest inadvertent facial nerve stimulation. No EMG responses were noted between the initial identification of the nerve and the close of surgery. On closure of the surgical site, the electrodes were removed and disposed of in the appropriate container. Postoperatively, the patient was noted to have complete and symmetrical facial movement.

Although this case describes a surgical procedure in which the intratemporal portion of the facial nerve is at risk for iatrogenic injury, essentially the same process and procedures are employed when either the intracranial or extratemporal portions of the nerve are at risk. Vigilance to EMG activity and correlation with surgical events are essential to a successful outcome. This vigilance is necessary whether the nerve is directly or indirectly at-risk for injury.

SUMMARY

IFNM provides a means of improving surgical efficacy in preserving facial nerve function postoperatively. A review by Harner, Daube, Ebersold and Beatty (1987) found that IFNM improved surgical efficacy in patients with acoustic neuromas. Gantz et al. (1982) evaluated the efficacy of IFNM in patients undergoing facial nerve decompression. IFNM enables identification of the site of conduction block in a majority of cases. A review of 250 mastoidectomies by Pensak et al. (1994) shows the efficacy of IFNM in identifying dehiscent or nonvisible facial nerves.

IFNM serves as an aid to a surgeon, but cannot serve as a replacement for sound clinical judgment. The surgeon integrates the information provided by IFNM with all other available information, including anatomical and surgical knowledge as well as visible landmarks within the surgical site, to make surgical decisions.

Given the possibility of equipment malfunction, technical error, or erroneous responses, facial nerve monitoring cannot replace proper surgical vigilance. Although the efficacy of IFNM has not been demonstrated for every surgical procedure for which the facial nerve is exposed or potentially at-risk for injury (Roland & Meyerhoff, 1993), some would argue that IFNM should be used in every otologic case (Silverstein, Rosenberg, Wilcox, & Gordon, 1994).

REFERENCES

Beck, D. L. (1993). Facial nerve electrophysiology: Electro-neurography and facial nerve monitoring. *Seminars in Hearing, 14,* 123–133.

Beck, D. L., Atkins, J. S., Benecke, J. E., & Brackmann, D. E. (1991). Intraoperative facial nerve monitoring: prognostic aspects during acoustic tumor removal. *Otolaryngology Head and Neck Surgery, 104,* 780–782.

Beck, D. L., & Benecke, J. E. (1990). Intraoperative facial nerve monitoring: Technical aspects. *Otolaryngology Head and Neck Surgery, 102,* 270–272.

Gantz, B. J., Gmur, A., & Fisch, U. (1982). Intraoperative evoked electromyography in Bell's Palsy. *American Journal of Otolaryngology, 3,* 273–278.

Harner, S. G., Daube, J. R., Ebersold, M. J., & Beatty, C. W. (1987). Improved preservation of facial nerve function with use of electrical monitoring during removal of acoustic neuromas. *Mayo Clinic Proceedings, 62,* 92–102.

Hogan, K. (1992). Neuroanesthetic techniques for intraoperative monitoring. In J. M. Kartusch & K. R. Bouchard (Eds.), *Neuromonitoring in otology and head and neck surgery* (pp. 61–79). New York: Raven Press.

Jacobson, G., & Tew, J. (1987). Intraoperative evoked potential monitoring. *Journal of Clinical Neurophysiology, 4,* 145–176.

Kartush, J. M. (1989). Electromyography and intraoperative facial monitoring in contemporary neurotology. *Otolaryngology Head and Neck Surgery. 101,* 496–503.

Kartush, J. M., & Bouchard, K. R. (1992). Intraoperative facial nerve monitoring: Otology, neurotology, and skull base surgery. In J. M. Kartusch & K. R. Bouchard (Eds.), *Neuromonitoring in otology and head and neck surgery* (pp. 99–120). New York: Raven Press.

Kartush, J. M., Niparko, J. K., Bledsoe, S. C., Graham, M. D., & Kemink, J. L. (1985). Intraoperative facial nerve monitoring: A comparison of stimulating electrodes. *Laryngoscope, 95,* 1536–1540.

May, M. (1986). Anatomy of the facial nerve for the clinician. In M. May (Ed.), *The facial nerve* (pp. 21–62). New York: Thieme Medical Publishers.

Moeller, A. R., & Janetta, P. J. (1984). Preservation of facial function during removal of acoustic neuromas. *Journal of Neurosurgery, 61,* 757–760.

Niparko, J. K., & Kileny, P. R. (1988). Intraoperative monitoring of facial function. *Seminars in Hearing, 9,* 127–139.

Pensak, M. L., Willging, J. P., & Keith, R. W. (1994). Intraoperative facial nerve monitoring in facial nerve surgery: A resident training experience. *American Journal of Otology, 15,* 108–110.

Prass, R. L. (1992). Intraoperative electromyographic recording. In J. M. Kartusch, & K. R. Bouchard (Eds.), *Neuromonitoring in otology and head and neck surgery* (pp. 81–97). New York: Raven Press.

Prass, R. L., & Luders, H. (1985). Constant-current versus constant-voltage stimulation. *Journal of Neurosurgery, 62,* 622–623.

Prass, R. L., & Luders, H. (1986). Acoustic (loudspeaker) facial electromyographic monitoring: Part one, evoked electromyographic activity during acoustic neuroma resection. *Neurosurgery, 19,* 392–400.

Roland, P. S., & Meyerhoff, W. L. (1993). Intraoperative facial nerve monitoring: What is its appropriate role? *American Journal of Otology, 14,* I.

Schwartz, D. M, Bloom, M. J., Pratt, R. E., & Costello, J. A. (1988). Anesthetic effects on neuroelectric events. *Seminars in Hearing, 9,* 99–112.

Schwartz, D. M. & Rosenberg, S. I. (1992). Facial nerve monitoring during parotidectomy. In J. M. Kartusch, & K. R. Bouchard (Eds.), *Neuromonitoring in otology and head and neck surgery* (pp. 121–130). New York: Raven Press.

Silverstein, H., Rosenberg, S. I., Wilcox, T. O., & Gordon, M. A. (1994). [Letter to the editor]. *American Journal of Otology, 15,* 121–122.

■ CHAPTER 5 ■

MONITORING THE COCHLEAR NERVE

■ DOUGLAS L. BECK, M.A. ■

The auditory brainstem response (ABR) is a physiologic event that occurs in response to stimulation of the ear. In the office, ABR serves two functions. The first is to estimate hearing sensitivity. This is useful when a patient is unable or unwilling to participate in standard behavioral audiometry. The second function of the ABR is to rule out (or evaluate) retrocochlear etiologies for an asymmetric, or anomalous hearing loss. In the operating room, ABR is used to monitor the status of the auditory system.

ABR has been scrutinized in the recent literature regarding sensitivity and selectivity (Wilson, Hodgson, Gustafson, Hogue, & Mills, 1992; Telian, Kileny, Niparko, Kemink, & Graham, 1989). ABR is highly effective in allowing the audiologist to estimate the degree and type of hearing loss objectively and continues to serve very well in the evaluation of retrocochlear hearing loss (Beck, 1993; Selters, 1993; Swan & Brown, 1989).

ABR serves a different function in the operating room. In the final analysis, intraoperative ABR can be thought of as "ABR maintenance." The goal is to maintain the ABR throughout the surgery.

Unfortunately, ABR is not a perfect test. In this respect it is in good company. Magnetic resonance imaging (MRI), computed tomography (CT), blood tests, physical examinations, and patients' recollections of their history are also not perfect.

It can be said that ABR is an objective test. However, for the ABR to be useful, someone needs to interpret it, and at that level, it becomes subjective.

It has been shown that despite normal hearing (or mild hearing loss), on rare occasions the ABR is not obtainable (Kraus, Ozdamar, Stein, & Reed, 1984; Starr et al., 1991). The reason for the absence of an ABR in an ear that appears to hear well is still unknown. It is important to realize that the ABR is not a hearing test.

ABR problems intensify and multiply in the operating room. During successful surgery, one expects the ABR to remain essentially intact. It is tempting to suggest that an unchanged ABR during surgery predicts unchanged hearing postoperatively. However, the ABR is not sensitive enough to detect all subtle changes the patient may notice or the postoperative audiogram may indicate. Likewise, intraoperative ABRs can be obliterated, yet the patient may have normal or unchanged hearing at the postoperative evaluation (Mustain, Al-Mefty, & Anand, 1992).

Typically, when the ABR is lost intraoperatively, the patient wakes up with additional hearing loss or a dead ear. This was recently described by Schwaber, Hall, and Zealer (1991) regarding the loss of both the electrocochleogram (ECoG) and the ABR during an acoustic neuroma removal surgery. Both auditory responses disappeared immediately following compromise of the vascular supply to the cochlea. The patient suffered complete and irreversible hearing loss on the affected side.

Other auditory evoked potentials are also used in the operating room. Direct nerve studies and ECoG add different yet complementary information to the intraoperative audiologic profile. These multiple modalities can be used individually or in tandem (Hall, Schwaber, Henry, & Baer, 1993; Kileny, Niparko, Shepard, & Kemink, 1988; Ruth, Mills, & Jane, 1986; Schwaber, et al., 1991), and will be discussed minimally in this chapter.

Example 1:
During a retrosigmoid vestibular nerve section, it is often appropriate to begin monitoring with ABR and ECoG. Once the surgeon has a direct view of the cochleovestibular nerve bundle, the surgeon may place an electrode on the cochlear nerve to determine which branch is cochlear and which is vestibular (referred to as a direct nerve study). This is easily determined because the vestibular branch will yield a minimal response (if at all) whereas the cochlear branch will yield a robust, triphasic, large amplitude response. Depending on the monitoring equipment used, the ABR, ECoG, and the direct nerve study can be obtained simultaneously.

In the above example, the ABR is essentially a gross overview of the auditory system, indicating neural synchrony and continuity. The direct nerve study yields a physiologic response which helps to define the anatomy. The ECoG reflects the status of the vascular system of the cochlea.

Although similar to standard clinical ABR, intraoperative ABR requires significant adaptation to be performed in the operating room. Flexibility and keen attention to detail are the primary components needed for successful intraoperative monitoring of the cochlear nerve.

Although some basic issues related to ABR are addressed, this chapter cannot suffice as a preliminary clinical introduction to ABR. Rather, it addresses the basic needs of the "operating room novice" in applying ABR knowledge to the operating room.

This chapter assumes that the novice has a working knowledge of ABR, and has performed at least 100 ABR evaluations in the office before attempting to perform an ABR in the operating room. The operating room is not a good place to learn how to perform an ABR evaluation. The reader is urged to master the clinical skills associated with ABR before entering the operating room. (See Jacobson and Balzar [1992] for a detailed discussion on this and other matters related to operating room concerns.)

ANATOMY

The auditory nerve (CN VIII) is a part of the combined vestibulocochlear nerve. The vestibulocochlear nerve carries two types of sensory information from the end organs to the brain. Hearing information is transmitted along the cochlear fibers and balance information is transmitted along the vestibular fibers. The auditory nerve is about 2.5 cm long. Each auditory nerve contains some 30,000 myelinated fibers (Moller, 1992a).

The vestibulocochlear nerve exits the ipsilateral brainstem immediately dorsal to the facial nerve. As the nerve approaches the medial end of the internal auditory canal (IAC) the auditory and vestibular fibers become distinguishable. At the brainstem, the two sets of fibers are intimately related.

Through the IAC, the vestibulocochlear nerve has three distinct branches—the superior vestibular nerve, the inferior vestibular nerve, and the cochlear nerve. Lateral to the IAC, the auditory nerve innervates the cochlea. The superior and inferior vestibular fibers innervate the semicircular canals.

The audiologist should know the anatomical landmarks relating to the middle ear, facial nerve, cochlea, semicircular canals, and CN VII and CN VIII in order to satisfactorily monitor the cochlear nerve (Figure 5-1). It is recommended that the audiologist spend time in the temporal bone lab, if possible. Observing ear surgery to become knowledgeable about the anatomy of the ear and the related neurological structures is an excellent way to learn the relevant anatomy.

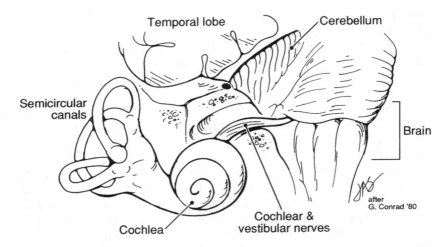

Temporal lobe   Cerebellum

Semicircular
canals

Brain

Cochlea   Cochlear &
vestibular nerves

after
G. Conrad '80

FIGURE 5–1. Basic inner ear anatomy.

THE AUDITORY BRAINSTEM RESPONSE: BASIC CONCEPTS

The ABR is a far-field response. We are not measuring directly from the neural generators, but are measuring a small electrical response using an electrode far away from the neurologic event itself.

Sophisticated computerized equipment and advanced protocols are used to identify and enhance the tiny amplitude responses buried deep within the avalanche of normal ongoing bioelectric activity (American Speech-Language-Hearing Association, 1988; Jewitt & Williston, 1971; Moller, 1992b; Ruth & Lambert, 1991).

The ABR typically has 5 to 7 peaks (Figure 5–2). These peaks are identified via signal averaging, amplification, common mode rejection, and appropriate filtering. The ABR has a high correlation to some aspects of hearing. However, an excellent ABR result does not guarantee the presence of normal hearing and normal hearing does not ensure that an ABR will be normal or even obtainable (Kraus et al., 1984; Starr et al., 1991). It is important to realize that an ABR is not a "hearing" test, rather, it is a test of neural synchrony.

APPROPRIATE CASES FOR ABR MONITORING

In essence, anytime intraoperative ABR monitoring is requested or anytime the patient's hearing is at risk during a surgical procedure, there is a valid

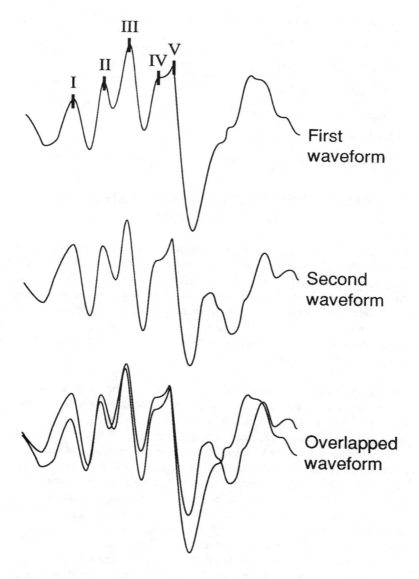

FIGURE 5–2. Normal ABR recording. Wave I = 1.7 msec, III = 3.8, V = 5.7.

reason to perform an intraoperative ABR. The most typical cases that are ABR monitored include:

Acoustic neuroma surgery with hearing preservation

Endolymphatic sac surgery

Vestibular nerve sections

Revision mastoid cases

Most posterior fossa cases

Microvascular decompressions

Others as requested by the surgeon

HEARING PRESERVATION, ABR, AND ACOUSTIC TUMOR REMOVAL

In July of 1988, magnetic resonance imaging (MRI) with gadolinium contrast became clinically available (Welling, Glasscock, Woods, & Jackson, 1990). This imaging technique revolutionized the detection of acoustic neuromas. As a result of this imaging milestone, small acoustic neuromas are being discovered and managed earlier than ever before. Tiny tumors can be found, and often removed before they destroy the patient's hearing. As such, hearing preservation has become more important than it was in the past (National Institutes of Health, 1991).

Unfortunately, only about one-third of the surgeries that attempt to preserve hearing are successful (Kveton, 1990). Among the issues addressed by the surgeon and the patient regarding tiny tumors in essentially asymptomatic patients are: Do the tiny tumors need to be removed? And, is the MRI with gadolinium 100% accurate in diagnosing tiny tumors?

A conservative approach might mandate observation and reevaluation once tumor growth is confirmed. Of course, once growth is confirmed in an appropriate patient, tumor removal should occur quickly. Removing smaller tumors is usually regarded as easier than removing larger tumors.

Regarding MRI accuracy, it is certainly the best imaging technique for acoustic tumors. However, MRI with gadolinium is not flawless. False–positive MRIs have been reported (von Glass, Haid, Cidlinski, Stenglein, & Christ, 1991; Welling et al., 1990). For the patient with normal hearing or only a mild sensorineural hearing loss and a small tumor (less than 1 cm), hearing preservation is a high priority. However, for the patient with a 3 cm tumor and an 85 dB hearing loss, hearing preservation is less of a priority. (See Chapter 11, Acoustic Neuroma Surgery, for a detailed discussion.)

Whether or not hearing preservation surgery is elected is a surgical decision made by the physician and the patient. The key factors in this decision have historically included "serviceable hearing" (often referred to as a speech reception threshold [SRT] of better than 50 dB and a word recognition score [WRS] of better than 50%), tumor size and location, risk of facial nerve injury, patient's age, medical history, general physical condition, and other factors.

In a recent paper on the prognostic factors related to hearing preservation in acoustic neuroma surgery, Shelton et al. (1989) noted a relationship between the preoperative interaural latency difference of the ABR wave V and hearing preservation. Specifically, they noted that when the interaural latency difference was less than 0.4 msec, 78% of the patients had postoperative hearing preservation. With an interaural wave V difference of between 0.5 msec and 2 msec, the preservation rate dropped to 58%; and when there was no response on the ABR, postoperative hearing was present in only half the patients.

Josey et al. (1988) also noted that the ABR was an important prognostic factor in hearing preservation. For patients with small tumors, intact residual hearing, good speech discrimination scores, normal acoustic reflexes, and good preoperative ABRs (waves I, III, and V identified), the success rate of hearing preservation was 68%.

Shelton, Hitselberger, House, and Brackmann (1990) evaluated the long-term results of hearing preservation in patients and discovered that 56% of the "preserved hearing" ears had significant hearing loss over the first 8 postoperative years. The question they addressed was: "Is preserved hearing after acoustic tumor removal sustained over time?" They conclude that there is a tendency for the preserved hearing in the operated ear to decline more quickly than the hearing in the nonoperated ear with respect to pure tones, SRT, and WRS. They state that hearing preservation should be pursued vigorously in appropriate patients. They note that their new criteria for hearing preservation surgery include an SRT of 30 dB or better and a WRS of 70% or better.

However, McKenna et al. (1992) report on 18 patients who had acoustic tumors removed via a suboccipital approach. Follow-up was as long as 10 years on some of the patients; 78% of the patients had no significant decline in the hearing of their operated ear.

STERILIZATION AND INFECTIOUS DISEASES

It is mandatory that all subdermal needle electrodes be appropriately sterilized. In general, anything coming in contact with the patient during surgery should be sterilized (Jacobson & Balzer, 1992), and whenever possible, should be discarded after use in the appropriate manner. Although some audiologists do not sterilize the stimulus delivery systems, it is recommended here. Decisions relating to sterilization techniques and protocols, materials, methods of choice, and related issues should be made with the physicians and the director of the operating rooms. The audiologist also should review the *Recommendations for Prevention of HIV Transmission in Health-Care Settings* by the Centers for Disease Control (1987).

Typically, ethylene oxide gas sterilization is used for sterilization of delicate components such as the stimulus delivery system. Autoclave (standard steam sterilization) techniques are fine for most subdermal needle electrodes. Manufacturers supply both presterilized parts and items that will need to be sterilized. The audiologist should read all manufacturers' instructions that accompany purchased parts to determine which items require sterilization and how to sterilize them. It is important to note that gas sterilization may take 24 hours or more. As such, sterilization decisions need to be discussed well in advance of the surgery to have the electrodes and other hardware ready in time for the operation.

PREOPERATIVE AUDIOLOGIC EVALUATION

It is important to have a complete preoperative audiometric evaluation and an ABR on all patients on whom an intraoperative ABR is to be attempted. It makes no sense to attempt to secure an intraoperative ABR without a complete assessment of the patient's hearing.

Severe and profound hearing losses will likely render the ABR useless. Mild-to-moderate sensorineural hearing losses may delay the latencies of an otherwise normal ABR. Patients with conductive and mixed losses present with delayed absolute latencies although the interpeak latencies may be essentially normal.

Abnormalities are best discovered during a routine audiometric evaluation and ABR performed preoperatively in the office rather than during surgery where anomalies may be misinterpreted as representative of an iatrogenic event.

The preoperative ABR is particularly important before an attempt to remove an acoustic neuroma with hearing preservation surgery. Not only is it important to determine the best stimulating and recording parameters preoperatively, but the ability to acquire an ABR may be an important factor in deciding whether to attempt hearing preservation (Josey, Glasscock, & Jackson, 1988; Shelton, Brackmann, House, & Hitselberger, 1989).

STIMULUS DELIVERY SYSTEMS

Standard headphone stimulus delivery systems are not useful in the operating room (Moller, 1992b). The majority of stimulus delivery systems used in the operating room involve some sort of "insert" earphone. Rather than placing an earphone on the ear, the earphone is placed in the ear.

Many types of inserts are available. Electrically driven, very small "button" receivers work fairly well. Button receivers are available at Radio Shack and similar electronic supply stores. A pair of button receivers costs about $12. An adapter cable is usually necessary to connect the button receiver to the output of the ABR equipment with adequate cable length. Twenty feet is about the length of cable necessary to allow flexibility and adequate equipment positioning. Twenty feet of extension cable costs less than $10.

Three-piece insert systems are available from most of the ABR equipment manufacturers at a cost of $300 to $500. The components include the transducer itself (approximately ¼ inch thick, 2 inches long and 1½ inches wide), a plastic sound transmission tube (approximately 10 inches in length) and the inserted spongy ear piece (similar to disposable noise protection kits).

Because the transducer and the recording electrodes are physically separated in the three-piece system, electromagnetic interference from the transducer is essentially eliminated from the ABR recording. Additionally, the spongy insert maintains and ensures a patent external auditory canal (see Figure 5–3).

Another option is to use a lucite ear mold "super glued" to the 10-inch tube and subsequently attached to the transducer. Lucite molds can be custom made or generically fit. When using a lucite mold in the ear canal, we use a surgical glue placed on the lucite ear mold (MASTISOL) to increase adhesion between the ear canal and the lucite mold. We have used this technique successfully on many occasions during vestibular nerve sections.

Whichever stimulus system is selected, additional anchoring is recommended to maintain the position of the stimulus delivery system in the ear canal. Inserts can be secured to the ear with tape, sutures, "bone wax," glues, and a variety of other methods. These can be used individually or in combination for added security. The security of the stimulus system within the ear canal cannot be overemphasized. This is the "weakest link" in the intraoperative ABR.

STIMULUS PARAMETERS

Our standard stimulating parameters for the office and in the operating room are:

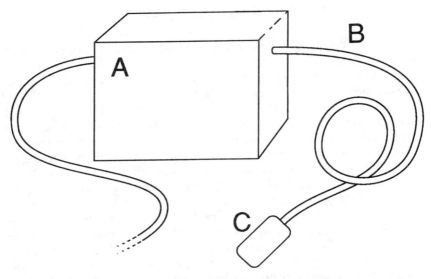

FIGURE 5–3. Insert ear system. A: Transducer, B: Plastic connector tube, C: Foamy ear insert.

PHASE: Rarefaction

RATE: 17.1 clicks per second

LOUDNESS: 90 dB

SAMPLE SIZE: 1500 clicks

If a repeatable, reliable ABR is obtained in the office using these parameters, the parameters are maintained in the operating room. If a good quality, repeatable ABR is not obtained, or if it is recently lost during surgery, the audiologist troubleshoots and adjusts the system as needed to interpret and report the problem and to produce the best possible ABR.

TROUBLESHOOTING ABRs

If, during surgery the ABR suddenly goes from a high quality, repeatable ABR to a series of poorly repeating bumps, immediate analysis and troubleshooting are initiated and a status report is given to the surgeon.

The first place to seek answers and rule out options is anesthesia. The audiologist should immediately consult with the anesthesiologist/anesthetist to determine if the anesthetic regimen, patient's temperature, or other anesthesiology controlled variables were recently altered. (For a complete discussion of these factors the reader is directed to Chapter 13, Anesthesia and Intraoperative Monitoring). Assuming that anesthesia cannot explain the ABR degradation, further analysis is undertaken.

The first "stimulus" parameter evaluated is the stimulus delivery system itself. This is particularly useful in the following surgical scenario:

EXAMPLE 2:
The intraoperative ABR has been fine and has repeated without problem throughout the case. The surgeon is not working near any auditory structures. However, the anesthesiologist has recently been working on the patient's airway, near the patient's mouth, under the sterile drapes. A few minutes later, the ABR is unobtainable.

This may indicate that the recording electrodes have been disconnected or damaged or that the stimulating system has been violated. These are known sources of intraoperative monitoring failure.

The electrodes can be assessed by performing an electrode impedance verification. High impedances may indicate the need for an electrode to be replaced (poor contact) or may be consistent with an open channel (dislodged electrode). When these situations occur in the operating room, the surgeon should be notified as soon as the anomaly is determined and a plan to manage the problem should be discussed.

The plan may include replacing the offending electrode or doing nothing, depending on where the surgeon is with respect to the cochlear nerve. The surgeon may feel that it is not worth the risk (to the sterile field) to fix the problem if he has already passed the point in the surgery where the cochlear nerve or blood supply were at risk. Likewise, he may decide to stop surgery immediately to replace the electrode.

If the ABR click is suddenly heard throughout the operating room, the likely problem is that the stimulating system has been dislodged from the ear or that a "disconnect" exists between the transducer and the ear. Again, the surgeon is notified and corrective action should be discussed. If repair is warranted, repair is undertaken cautiously, with respect to sterile technique, if and when the surgeon feels it is appropriate to do so.

In these situations, the surgeon must be informed immediately of the problem. It is inappropriate to allow the surgeon to think that intraoperative monitoring is occurring when, in fact, an electrode went bad or a similar failure occurred some time ago.

In this author's experience, the rule of thumb in most operating rooms is "no news is good news." That is, the anesthesiologist will not announce the patient's latest vitals, unless there is a problem. Likewise, the circulating nurse will not announce to the entire operating room which required instruments were just brought into the room (unless they are late and the surgeon is waiting). If the audiologist does not announce a problem, the surgeon will probably assume everything is all right.

STIMULUS PARAMETER VARIABLES

If the problem is not readily detectable and repairable, the audiologist should announce the problem to the surgeon and attempt software changes to correct the problem. The audiologist will need to alter the ABR stimulating and recording parameters in a manner similar to the approach taken in the office to "clean up" or better define the ABR.

RATE OF PRESENTATION

Decreasing the rate of the stimulus should decrease the latencies of the ABR and should produce better overall morphology. This is thought to result from an increase in neural synchrony. Typically, if 17.1 clicks per second does not yield a good result, 11.1 clicks per second may be attempted. Certainly one can present slower than 11.1, perhaps 7.1 or so, but the problem is that decreasing the ABR click rate (although likely to produce a better waveform) slows down the analysis and interpretation time. ABR is most useful during surgery when it can be quickly and accurately obtained and interpreted.

Although a minute or two in the office is not an excessively long analysis and interpretation time, in the operating room, it is. The real time involved to obtain 1500 clicks at 17.1 per second is 1.5 minutes. The real time elapsed at 7.1 clicks per second is 3.5 minutes. The extra 2 minutes can be an epic adventure in stress and anxiety when the surgeon is waiting for a response to the question, "How's the hearing?", particularly after cauterizing a few small, unidentified bleeders.

SAMPLE SIZE

Regarding sample size, it is not necessary to complete the entire series of 1500 clicks. For example, if a clear waveform is identified at approximately 750 clicks, this may be acceptable depending on the task at hand. A recent clinical paper endorses using smaller sample sizes and discontinuing the test once the wave is identified. The proposed sample size was between 500 and 750 clicks (Beattie, Zipp, Schaffer, & Silzel, 1992).

The primary advantage of the more traditional (larger) sample size is to reduce biologic background noise. During surgery, physiologic background noise is greatly reduced secondary to the patient being asleep and anesthetized. Therefore, background noise is less of a factor with intraoperative ABR than with clinical ABR, and one can extrapolate that using a smaller sample size may be reasonable.

LOUDNESS

Another option to improve the ABR is to make the signal louder. Just as slowing down the click rate increases the amplitude and decreases the latencies of the ABR, this can also be accomplished by increasing the loudness of the stimulus. There is an inverse relationship between loudness and latency. As loudness increases, latency decreases. This relationship allows the ABR to be used to approximate auditory thresholds (see Figure 5–4).

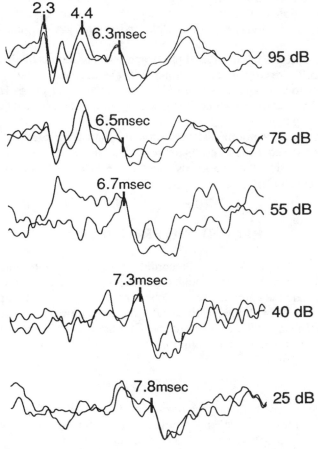

FIGURE 5–4. Latency versus loudness function.

PHASE

Changing the phase of the stimulus (alternating, rarefaction or condensation) may improve the quality of the ABR, particularly in cases of high-frequency hearing losses. However, one should try to maintain the same phase throughout the procedure whenever possible. If an intraoperative event attenuates or eliminates the ABR, and if the ABR can be improved by a change in the stimulation phase, then the interpretation of the newly improved data is somewhat awkward.

It is known that, when patients with normal hearing are tested in the office, polarity is of little consequence with respect to threshold analysis (Sininger & Masuda, 1990).

Clinically, it appears that the selection of phase is probably less important than the adherence to a specific phase. One should not mix a left ear ABR using rarefaction with a right ear ABR using condensation. Likewise, starting a case with rarefaction and finishing with condensation is a less than desirable protocol.

Rarefaction is the most used phase and condensation is likely the least used phase. There is evidence that some types and degrees of hearing loss are more likely to be evaluated successfully using a particular phase. However, this should be determined clinically in the preoperative assessment before the start of the operation.

With respect to normal listeners, standard clinical ABR tests using click stimuli produce equivalent results for condensation and rarefaction. (For an excellent discussion of phase and its effect on the ABR, the reader is urged to read Fowler [1992]).

RECORDING PROTOCOLS

A standard 3-lead, single channel recording system is typical for intraoperative ABR recordings. Vertex (or high forehead) is positive, ipsilateral ear lobe is negative, and the contralateral ear lobe serves as reference. This protocol produces an ABR with the positive peaks displayed upwards, as is the convention in the United States. Two channel paradigms can be used but are not advocated for intraoperative monitoring by the beginner.

CUP ELECTRODES

Cup electrodes are not favored in the operating room. When they are used in the operating room they are rarely sterilized. Most often they are cleaned with alcohol. This is probably adequate because cup electrodes typically do not come in contact with bodily fluids. However, if cup electrodes are "contaminated," appropriate cleaning and sterilization is in order before re-use.

Standard cup electrodes can be used in the operating room if they are not in the way of the surgical field and if they maintain appropriate impedances and adhesion throughout the case.

When using cup electrodes, surgical tape is placed over the bowl of the cup electrode to increase adhesion. Surgical tape or collodion may be used to increase adhesion. Although this works reasonably well, collodion is toxic and flammable. Extreme caution is required.

Cup electrodes require an electrolyte gel to serve as an interface between the electrode and the skin. The gel can dry out during long procedures. This is "diagnosed" by an increase in recording electrode impedances with no other apparent reason. If this were to occur during a surgical procedure, it would be difficult (occasionally impossible) to fix the problem because access to the recording electrodes is often impossible once surgery has started.

The tape used to provide extra adhesion for cup electrodes may also be problematic as it occupies valuable space within the surgical field. Further, tape tends to loosen, and adhesion will lessen as the tape gets wet or occasionally saturated.

During most otologic, neurotologic, and neurosurgical cases the patient's head is covered by sterile drapes, sterile tapes, sterile plastics, sterile irrigation tubes, anesthesia equipment, and numerous surgical items rendering the head essentially inaccessible in all but a few cases. This complete draping of the patient's head renders cup electrodes less than adequate as they are not available for adjustment once surgery has started. It is prudent to minimize the need for intraoperative adjustments of the equipment.

DISPOSABLE SUBDERMAL NEEDLE ELECTRODES

Disposable subdermal needle electrodes are the preferred electrodes (Keith & Bankaitis, 1993). They are inexpensive, quick and easy to insert, and the safest option for all concerned (when disposed of properly). All needle electrodes must be sterilized prior to use. One must follow the manufacturer's advice on how to clean and sterilize the electrodes. Some manufacturers recommend soaking the electrodes in a Clorox solution before sterilization. As noted above, some manufacturers offer presterilized, disposable subdermal needle electrodes.

Due to the very small surface area of the subdermal needle electrode, there is a minimal risk of electrical burns to the patient in the event of a "ground" failure. It is extremely rare for such an event to happen (Moller, 1992b).

Needle electrodes are obtainable through the major ABR equipment manufacturers and other sources. Needle electrodes are the most popular type of recording electrodes used in the operating room for intraoperative ABR.

Subdermal needle electrodes placed within the pinna's lobule are easily placed and present very little risk to the patient. It is rare for any significant bleeding to occur as a result of placing an electrode in the lobule. It is useful to bend the tip of the electrode into a right angle before placing the electrode in the lobule. This provides an "anchor" and helps to ensure that the electrode will not be accidentally dislodged. Nonetheless, it is a good idea to place tape on the electrode hub and along the wire to add "strain relief" (see Figure 5-5).

When placing electrodes and securing the hardware it is important to verify that the monitoring equipment is not in the surgical field and that it does not prevent the surgeon from gaining the needed exposure. It is also important to choose a recording site as close as possible to the neural generator site (the cochlea or distal end of the VIIIth nerve).

Our typical recording sites are:

Vertex (CZ)   Positive (noninverting)
Ipsilateral ear lobe   Negative (inverting)
Contralateral ear lobe Reference

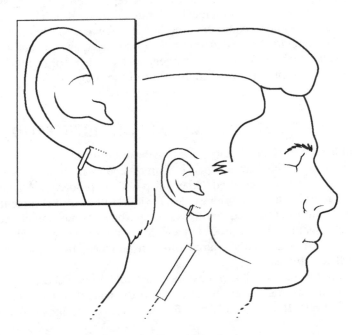

FIGURE 5-5. Subdermal needle electrode within the inferior pinna.

HEAD BOX

The unit the electrodes are plugged into is referred to as the "head box." In a standard otologic case, the head box is placed to the right of the patient for a left ear case and to the left of the patient for a right ear case. The exact location is not critical and the audiologist must remain flexible because the same location will not always be available.

The primary factors to address when placing the headbox are that the head box should be accessible, secure, and protected from fluids. The head box should be taped and draped to secure and protect it as needed. Some equipment manufacturers have special "surgical head boxes" which are useful in reducing or eliminating electromagnetic interference. These are useful and recommended here.

IMPEDANCES

Subdermal needle electrodes typically will yield impedances between 5000 and 10,000 ohms. Not only is the absolute impedance value important, but the "balancing" of the electrodes is also important. If all of the electrodes measured between 2000 and 3000 ohms, this would be very good. However, if two of the electrodes are determined to be between 1000 and 2000 ohms, and the third electrode is at 8000 ohms, this represents an imbalance, despite all of the values being less than 10,000 ohms.

In this situation, the high impedance electrode should be removed, perhaps cleaned with alcohol, and re-inserted. If the electrode continues to demonstrate a high impedance, it should be discarded in the "sharps" box, and replaced with a new, sterile electrode.

RECORDING PARAMETERS

Our standard recording parameters are:

Low pass filter at 1500 Hz

High pass filter at 150 Hz

15 msec window

10 microvolt sensitivity

Using the above mentioned 15 msec window, rather than the standard 10 msec window, allows more analysis time to be packed into the same space. The result is better definition of the ABR peaks, and an easier task when attempting to follow a given peak, such as wave V.

The majority of papers addressing ABR mention filter settings of about 150 Hz (high pass) to about 3000 Hz (low pass). However, using a low pass of 1500 Hz usually results in a less noisy recording with clearer peaks (Cacace, Shy, & Satya-Murti, 1980; Moller, 1987) (see Figure 5-6).

RECORDING ELECTRODE PLACEMENT

Before the needle is inserted through the skin, the recording electrode sites are cleaned using an alcohol-soaked cotton ball or pledget. The subdermal needle electrode is bent to a 90° angle and inserted into the prepared site. The electrode wires are braided together to reduce the likelihood of interference and secured out of the way with tape.

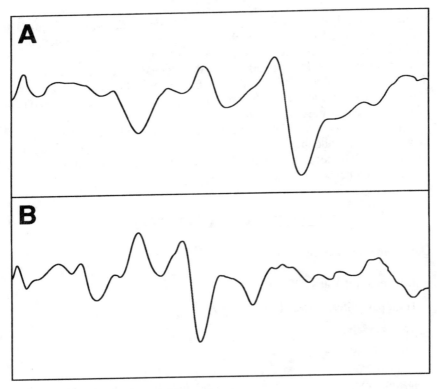

FIGURE 5-6.   A; 10 msec window ABR. B; 15 msec window ABR.

PREOPERATIVE EQUIPMENT SETUP

It is important to carefully think through and write down the steps involved in setting up the recording and stimulating equipment in the operating room. Once the patient has been intubated, things occur quickly. Setting up the patient should take less than 5 minutes and should be successful the first time.

The 5-minute window seems significantly shorter when you are first starting out and the entire operating room staff is watching, perhaps whispering, and waiting for you to finish so the surgeon can start the procedure. You must know all of the steps in order and execute them quickly and efficiently. Rehearsing the steps verbally with a trusted colleague is a good idea.

On entering the operating room, locate the best place for the ABR computer with respect to the position of the patient and the best available wall outlet. Preferably, the ABR computer should be plugged into an outlet without other equipment. Turn on the computer and boot up the ABR program. Start and complete all of the hardware and software preparation before the patient is brought into the operating room.

Confirm that the preoperative hearing test and the preoperative ABR are in the operating room for use as a reference. Make sure that the sterile insert stimulus delivery system, a back-up unit, surgical tape, and at least twice the number of sterile electrodes anticipated are ready.

Confirm that alcohol pledgets or alcohol-soaked cotton balls are ready and waiting. The head box cable should be plugged into the ABR computer and the head box should be secured to the operating room table. (See Figure 5–7 for the recommended operating room setup.)

PREOPERATIVE PATIENT PREPARATION

Sterile technique must be used when setting up the patient. I "scrub" and wear sterile surgical gloves while preparing the patient and hooking up the recording and stimulating equipment to the patient. Once the anesthesiologist has secured the airway, ask the anesthesiologist if it is all right to proceed. Once permission is obtained, start working on the patient.

Unwrap three previously sterilized, color-coded, subdermal needle electrodes and place a 90° angle between the hub and the needle point on each electrode. This is accomplished by holding the needle hub in one hand while gently but firmly bending the needle over with the index finger of the other hand to approximate a right angle.

Use the alcohol-soaked pledget (or cotton) to clean the intended recording sites immediately before insertion. A few gentle yet generous strokes

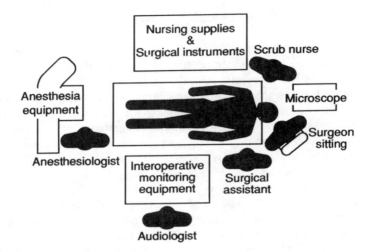

FIGURE 5–7. Operating room setup.

of the alcohol pledget across the insertion site are usually all that is required for adequate cleansing.

The needle electrodes are placed within the target tissue. The color-coded wires make tracing the wire from the recording site to the head box easy in case of an electrode failure. Tape placed over the electrode hub and along the wire helps to ensure that the electrode will not be accidentally removed.

The electrode wires are routed away from the surgical site, braided when possible and taped securely to the patient or the table to hold the wires in place and to add "strain relief" in case they are accidentally tugged.

The electrode wires are plugged into the head box under the table. Impedances are immediately verified to be within the target range (less than 10,000 ohms of impedance and less than 3000 ohms variance across all electrodes).

If there is a chance of fluid contacting the head box, a plastic liner is taped over the head box to serve as an "umbrella-like" layer of protection. In this way, fluid is diverted away from the head box.

As soon as the recording electrodes are inserted, an impedance check is performed. Once the impedance check is completed, and the values are determined to be acceptable, the previously sterilized transducer is placed in the ear canal. (Whether the ear canal is cleaned, prepped, and dried prior to the transducer placement is the surgeon's decision. For mastoid cases, the surgeon will probably want the ear canal to be prepped in case the canal is violated. However, for a retrosigmoid vestibular nerve section, the canal may not need to be prepped. This is the surgeon's decision and should be discussed ahead of time.)

The transducer needs to be secured vigorously so the surgical manipulations do not dislodge the unit. Place the insert in the canal, place sterile "bone wax" around the perimeter of the transducer and across the back of the transducer, and finally tape the transducer in place across the pinna. Other methods of securing the system to the ear are acceptable. It is recommended that these be discussed with the surgeon ahead of time.

Notify the surgeon that the "ear-piece" is the weakest link in the ABR chain and it needs to be moved and manipulated gently. The surgical manipulation of the pinna ("pinna retraction") during postauricular approaches to the ear may cause problems for ABR monitoring.

The typical problem is that the transducer is dislodged from the ear canal when the pinna is mobilized. If the transducer is dislodged, it reduces the sound pressure level of the click and attenuates or eliminates the ABR recording.

Once the insert is placed and secured, the first postintubation/preoperative baseline ABRs are obtained. In some respects the ABR obtained at this point is the easiest one to obtain. The preoperative ABR evaluation can be used to determine the starting stimulation parameters. The patient will likely have no muscle artifact because of muscle relaxants used for intubation and the overall sedative action of the anesthesia.

BASELINE ABR

A minimum of two ABR traces should be obtained. If they are identical with respect to waves I, III, and V latencies and grossly repeatable with respect to the overall morphology, then an adequate "baseline ABR" has been established. If the ABR traces vary, a third or fourth trace should be obtained to establish the true baseline. If a baseline is not forthcoming, troubleshooting must immediately be undertaken. The audiologist cannot afford to waste time on the fifth or sixth trace as the starting time of the true surgical procedure gets closer with every passing minute.

NON-AUDITORY REASONS FOR ABR VARIATIONS

The most important nonauditory factor that can alter the ABR during surgery is anesthesia. Although the ABR is known to be "relatively pharmacologically resistant," even commonly used anesthetics will increase latencies or reduce amplitude when used in larger concentrations. Among these anesthetic agents are enflurane, halothane, and isoflurane. (See Chapter 13, for a thorough discussion.)

Another factor that can affect the ABR is temperature. As the patient's body cools, the ABR latencies increase and the amplitudes decrease. During open heart procedures, the patient is intentionally cooled to stop the heart, reduce blood flow, reduce the brain's need for oxygenated blood, and slow metabolic functions. As can be seen in Figure 5–8, temperature is a variable that needs to be monitored by the audiologist, especially during long surgical procedures.

"Neural dysynchronization" can cause total obliteration of the ABR, as will be demonstrated later in Case Study 1. In essence, inadvertent mechanical manipulation of the cochlear nerve can eliminate the ABR, probably due to a synchronous conduction of the nerve impulse as it travels from the cochlea, along CN VIII, to the cochlear nuclei. In these instances, it is almost

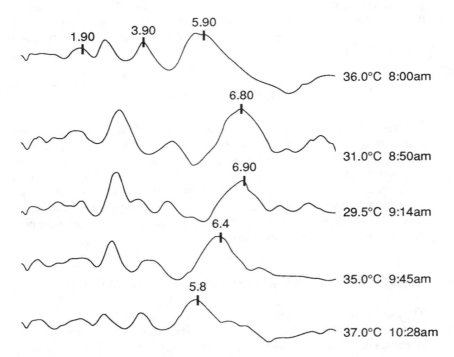

FIGURE 5–8. Latency versus temperature function.

impossible to determine the cause of the problem accurately or the likely outcome with respect to the patient's hearing.

Drilling on the mastoid bone during surgery may cause a temporary threshold shift or a permanent change in the patient's hearing. Drilling may be as brief as a few minutes in a revision case, but may endure for 4 or 5 hours in some cases. If the sound pressure level at the cochlea is sufficient to cause a change in the sensitivity of the ear (permanent or temporary), the ABR may be attenuated or eliminated.

As mentioned above, the transducer is the weakest link in the ABR stimulation system. If the transducer works its way out of the ear canal, or if the canal fills with fluid (irrigation fluid, blood, cerebrospinal fluid), or if the transducer fails, these events look very much like a damaged auditory system.

It is very difficult to rule out transducer problems during surgery. Unfortunately, many of the same attributes that are consistent with transducer failures (reduced amplitude and increased latencies) are also consistent with a compromised blood supply to the auditory system and an iatrogenically sectioned cochlear nerve.

WHAT IS A SIGNIFICANT CHANGE IN THE ABR?

One of the most important questions for the audiologist in the operating room is "What is a significant change in the ABR?" Unfortunately, the answer is highly elusive. There are general guidelines that can be applied, but the reader is advised to discuss this most important issue with the surgeon well in advance of the surgery.

If intraoperative monitoring were to be boiled down to its essence, we would find that the primary goals are to monitor the status of the auditory system and to alert the surgeon to physiologic changes as early as possible. If one waits too long before reporting changes, the etiology of the change may become irreversible.

On the other hand, if one reports every miniscule change, particularly when the surgeon is nowhere near the structure at issue, the audiologist may be thought to be a dolt and the monitoring subsequently ignored.

Knowing how and when to report changes in the ABR is somewhat subjective. When this information is managed and delivered efficiently and effectively, it is highly valued. When it is delivered late, or in a confusing manner it has no value at all. The following are ABR events reported as being associated with "unfavorable outcomes" (Jacobson, 1993).

Decrease in wave I-wave V interwave interval due to an increase in wave I latency.

Loss of all components beyond wave I or waves I and II.

Loss of wave V.

50% (or more) loss of any ABR component.

Loss of any ABR component.

Loss of the ABR.

Abrupt loss of the ABR.

Worsening AP (recorded from promontory).

Jacobson reports that there are no universally accepted "warning criteria." Jacobson refers to Moller's suggestion that it is probably prudent to advise the surgical team of any observed "negative trends," regardless of the magnitude.

CASE STUDY 1

A 38-year-old male roofer presented with a 2-month history of spinning vertigo, fluctuating low-frequency hearing loss, and tinnitus in the left ear. The otologist diagnosed Meniere's disease. The patient was medically treated for 2 months, but the symptoms persisted. The otologist suggested an endolymphatic sac shunt as a probable surgical cure, stating the cure rate with the "sac" procedure to be about 65 or 70%. The patient indicated he would rather elect a procedure with a higher "cure" rate and the retrosigmoid vestibular nerve section was discussed. The patient agreed to the risks and complications and underwent the procedure.

During the procedure, intraoperative facial nerve monitoring was used in tandem with intraoperative ABR and ECoG. At the ready was a cotton wick electrode, which could be placed directly on the cochlear and vestibular nerves in case physiologic identification of the vestibular fibers was required (Moller, 1987).

The facial nerve monitor indicated essentially a quiet baseline maintained throughout the case. The EMG baseline was within normal limits at 19 microvolts (Beck & Benecke, 1990). An excellent, robust contraction was observed (1200 microvolts) using 0.05 mA monopolar stimulus (Beck, Atkins, Brackmann, & Benecke, 1991) before and after the nerve sectioning.

The ABR baseline was obtained after the patient had been intubated and the baseline recording was repeated and verified. While establishing the surgical plane to identify the vestibular portion of the VIIIth nerve, the ABR latencies increased significantly and the ABR amplitude decreased. The audiologist reported this information to the surgeon.

A few minutes later, as the neurosurgeon was preparing to section the vestibular portion of the nerve, the ABR was essentially lost. The ECoG remained intact. This information was relayed to the surgeon.

The surgeon placed the cotton wick electrode on the cochlear nerve, producing a robust (33 microvolt), tri-phasic waveform; and the audiologist reported this finding as consistent with the cochlear division. The surgeon then placed the same electrode on the suspected vestibular nerve bundle and the audiologist reported the amplitude as 25% of the previously reported cochlear amplitude, with poor morphology. The surgeon decided that the direct nerve study confirmed which nerve bundle contained the vestibular fibers and the vestibular nerve was sectioned. On completion of the nerve section, the cotton wick electrode was again placed on the suspected cochlear nerve and the presection amplitude was confirmed.

During replacement of the bone flap, the ABR reappeared. By the time the last suture was placed, the ABR approximated the preoperative baseline recording.

Two weeks after surgery the patient returned to the office for a postoperative evaluation. The patient's hearing was unchanged as evidenced by the postoperative audiogram. The patient's facial function was normal. The patient reported complete relief from his presenting symptoms.

Case Study 1 illustrates the contributions of the additional cochlear nerve monitoring protocols, specifically, direct nerve monitoring and the ECoG. Unfortunately, this case also illustrates the lack of reliability of the intraoperative ABR when used exclusively. If the surgeon had stopped the case and had not sectioned the nerve based on the loss of the ABR, this would have been a mistake as evidenced by the postoperative hearing result.

The surgeon felt confident that the vascular supply to the cochlea was intact as the ECoG remained essentially unchanged. Further, the surgeon believed that the cochlear and the vestibular fibers were adequately identified and confirmed by using the direct nerve study. Specifically, the audiologist reported a much greater amplitude and the typical tri-phasic waveform when the cotton wick electrode was placed on the suspected auditory fibers. Likewise, a clearly attenuated response was noted from the suspected vestibular fibers.

This case also points out one of the many dilemmas that occur with intraoperative monitoring. That is, when the physiologic data contradict the anatomical data, which one is relied upon? The answer varies with the surgeon's experience, the audiologist's experience, the quality of the data, and many related factors (see Figure 5–9).

CASE STUDY 2

A 45-year-old female presented with an 8-month history of right-sided unilateral tinnitus. Her audiogram revealed a mild high-frequency hearing

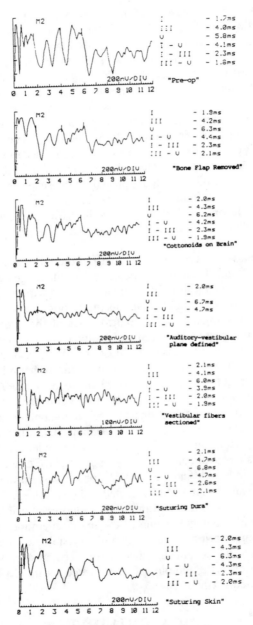

FIGURE 5-9. Intraoperative ABR changes from normal, to nondetectable, to normal.

loss in the right ear with normal hearing in the left ear. She reported no other auditory or otologic complaints. An ABR was ordered. It revealed a 0.7 msec interaural difference in wave V. An MRI with gadolinium was ordered, and it revealed a 6 mm vestibular schwannoma (acoustic neuroma) in the medial end of the internal auditory canal.

The otologist and the patient decided to observe the tumor over time. A repeat MRI was obtained 3 months later and tumor growth was confirmed. The second MRI revealed a 1.5 cm tumor that minimally extended into the cerebellopontine angle.

A middle fossa approach was elected to attempt hearing preservation. The patient was scheduled for surgery 1 week later. An ear impression was taken by the audiologist, of the right ear, and sent to the lab to have a lucite, deep canal, full-shell ear mold made. When the ear mold arrived 3 days later, the audiologist "super-glued" the 10-inch tube to the ear mold, and had the unit (tube and earmold) gas sterilized for use in the operating room.

After successful endotracheal intubation, the recording electrodes were attached to the patient by the audiologist. The impedances were confirmed. The surgeon elected to clean the ear with Betadine and dried the ear with sterile surgical cotton swabs before placing the sterile lucite ear-piece in the ear canal. As he placed the ear mold, he applied Mastisol to the ear mold to ensure a tight fit with excellent adhesion.

While the baseline ABR was being obtained, the facial nerve monitoring equipment was attached. The integrity of the facial nerve system was verified and the second ABR was obtained. The two preoperative ABRs confirmed each other and a "nonstimulus" trial was obtained. The nonstimulus trial serves to confirm that the ABR obtained is in fact different from the ongoing electrical activity. (Non-stimulus trials are useful when the ABR becomes ambiguous and questions of acoustic stimulation, neural injury, anesthesia-related changes, and other factors are considered in order to analyze the diminished ABR.)

As the surgeon drilled away the internal auditory canal, the ABR amplitude was attenuated. Rather than the full complement of waves that were identified on the preoperative ABR, only a small amplitude wave V remained. The audiologist reported this to the surgeon. The surgeon adjusted the retractor used to push away the brain, and the ABR returned to approximately the preoperative values. As the surgeon started to remove tumor from the auditory nerve, the ABR was lost.

The surgeon was able to visualize the root entry zone of CN VIII at the brainstem and felt confident that the nerve was intact. The audiologist conferred with the anesthesiologist to see if the anesthetic regimen had changed in the last few minutes. The anesthesiologist reported no changes. The audiologist verified the electrode impedances and increased the loudness of the

ABR click to the maximum output (99 dB). The presentation rate was slowed to 9.1 clicks per second, but again, the ABR was unobtainable.

The surgeon was updated on the ABR and the troubleshooting procedure the audiologist had already instituted. The audiologist suggested that if the surgeon was able to, it could be useful to place a finger over the transducer to determine that it was in its original preoperative position. A few minutes later when the tumor had been completely removed, the surgeon pressed the transducer into the ear canal, holding it tightly in position. The surgeon requested that another ABR be attempted. The audiologist ran an ABR and reported that waves I and III were apparent, although attenuated. As the surgeon closed the wound, the ABR amplitude increased and the waveform became repeatable. The audiologist informed the surgeon that the ABR suggested probable postoperative hearing.

Two weeks postoperatively, the patient was tested in the office and a 40 dB hearing loss was noted in the operated ear. The word recognition score of the operated ear was reported as 76%.

ELECTROCOCHLEOGRAPHY (ECoG)

Although the focus of this chapter is applying ABR to intraoperative monitoring, it is appropriate to give some attention to ECoG, as it, too, is used to monitor the auditory system during surgery. ECoG is typically used with ABR in surgeries that place the auditory system at risk for iatrogenic insult (Ferraro, 1993).

In essence, the ECoG action potential (AP) is wave I of the ABR. The ECoG yields specific and sensitive information regarding the most peripheral component of the auditory system (Ruth, Lambert, & Ferraro, 1988). The most likely information that the ECoG provides intraoperatively relates to the status of the cochlea and its vascular supply. Schwaber et al. (1991) note that the cessation of blood flow to the cochlea is usually associated with loss of wave I within 30 seconds.

The click stimulus used to elicit the ABR is essentially the same stimulus used to elicit the ECoG. (However, alternating clicks are the preferred phase for ECoG.) Slight variations in the recording protocol allow the more specific ECoG to be maximized.

Recording electrodes are of two types: extratympanic (indicating that the recording electrode is lateral to the eardrum), and transtympanic (indicating that the electrode is placed through the eardrum by the surgeon) and rests on the promontory or the round window.

Transtympanic electrodes (needle or ball end) allow the recording of very large amplitude potentials, requiring almost no averaging. Latencies for the transtympanic or extratympanic procedures are essentially the same.

In the office, ECoG is examined in terms of the action potential and the summating potential (SP). The SP:AP ratio is an analysis of amplitude that may indicate the presence of endolymphatic hydrops, consistent with Meniere's disease.

It is tempting to assume that, if the previously abnormal (positive) SP:AP ratio is representative of cochlear hydrops, or Meniere's disease, and the ratio "normalizes" during an endolymphatic sac surgery, this "normal" intraoperative ECoG is consistent with a "cure." Unfortunately, the author has seen this phenomenon a number of times in patients who have gone on to have a vestibular nerve section at a later date (indicating that the cure did not happen, or was temporary). There are no known large studies of this aspect of cochlear nerve monitoring in a peer reviewed journal, which have evaluated this issue.

A very important consideration when using the ECoG is to realize that it is not immediately sensitive to cochlear nerve injury. Ruth, Lambert, and Ferraro (1988) noted that, in humans, a wave I response when measured at the promontory remained unchanged for 25 minutes following an auditory nerve section. They also reported that a patient who was deafened intraoperatively maintained a wave I response for over 8 days.

Clearly, even a well functioning cochlea that has been disconnected from the brain will not hear. The cochlea may emit a neurophysiologic response, but if the VIIIth nerve is sectioned, hearing will not occur. It seems likely that an ECoG response can be obtained even in the absence of postoperative hearing.

CONCLUSION

Intraoperative cochlear nerve monitoring is an evolving science. As such, it is not perfect. Intraoperative ABR, even when performed flawlessly, can demonstrate false positives and false negatives.

Most audiologists combine intraoperative cochlear nerve monitoring protocols in order to better understand the relationship between the surgery and its effect on the patient's hearing.

There are as of yet no published, controlled studies that compare monitored to unmonitored patients with respect to hearing preservation and intraoperative decision making.

Once the audiologist has reported the intraoperative results to the surgeon, it is up to the surgeon to decide the value of the information and to act accordingly.

REFERENCES

American Speech-Language-Hearing Association, (1988). ASHA Working Group. *The short latency auditory evoked potentials.* [Tutorial] Rockville, MD: Author.

Beattie, R. C., Zipp, J. A., Schaffer, C. A., & Silzel, K. L. (1992). Effects of sample size on the latency and amplitude of the auditory evoked response. *American Journal of Otology, 13* (1), 55–67.

Beck, D. L. (1993). Auditory brainstem response testing (Letter to the editor). *Laryngoscope, 103* (5). 579–580.

Beck D. L., & Benecke, J. E. (1990). Intraoperative facial nerve monitoring: Technical aspects. *Otolaryngology—Head and Neck Surgery, 102* (3), 270–272.

Beck, D. L., Atkins, J. Brackmann, D. E., & Benecke, J. E. (1991). Intraoperative facial nerve monitoring: Prognostic aspects. *Otolaryngology—Head and Neck Surgery, 104* (6), 780–782.

Cacace, A. T., Shy, M., & Satya-Murti. (1980). Brainstem auditory evoked potentials: A comparison of two high-frequency filter settings. *Neurology, 30,* 765–767.

Centers for Disease Control. (1987, August). Acquired immunodeficiency syndrome, AIDS: Recommendations and guidelines. Atlanta, GA: Centers for Disease Control, Public Health Service, Dept. of Health and Human Services.

Ferraro, J. A. (1993). Electrocochleography: Clinical applications. *Audiology Today, 5* (6), 36–38.

Fowler, C. G. (1992). Effects of stimulus phase on the normal auditory brainstem response. *Journal of Speech and Hearing Research, 35* (2), 167–174.

Hall, J. W., Schwaber, M. K., Henry, M. M., & Baer, J. E. (1993). Intraoperative monitoring of the auditory system for hearing preservation. *Seminars in Hearing, 14* (2), 143–154.

Jacobson, G. P. (1993, Winter). The warning: How much change is too much change? *The Monitor* (The American Society of Neurophysiologic Monitoring), *1* (1), 5–6.

Jacobson, G. P., & Balzar, G. K. (1992) Basic considerations in intraoperative monitoring: Working in the operating room. J. Kartush & K. Bouchard (Eds.), *Neuromonitoring in otology and head and neck surgery* (pp. 21–60). Raven Press.

Jewitt, D. L., & Williston, J. S. (1971). Auditory evoked far fields averaged from the scalp of humans. *Brain, 94,* 681–696.

Josey, A. F., Glasscock, M. E., & Jackson, C. G. (1988). Preservation of hearing in acoustic tumor surgery: Audiologic indicators. *Annals of Otology, Rhinology and Laryngology, 97,* 626–630.

Keith, R. W., & Bankaitis, A. E. (1993). Intraoperative monitoring of the auditory brainstem response and facial nerve. *Current Opinions In Otolaryngology & Head and Neck Surgery, 1,* 64–71.

Kileny, P. R., Niparko, J. K., Shepard, N. T., & Kemink, J. L. (1988). Neurophysiologic intraoperative monitoring: l. Auditory function. *The American Journal of Otology, 9* (Supp.), 17–24.

Kraus, N., Ozdamar, O., Stein, L., & Reed, N. (1985). Absent auditory brainstem response: Peripheral hearing loss or brainstem dysfunction? *Laryngoscope, 94* (3), 400–406.

Kveton. J. F. (1990). Delayed spontaneous return of hearing after acoustic tumor surgery: Evidence for cochlear nerve conduction block. *Laryngoscope, 100,* 473–476.

McKenna, M. J., Halpin, C., Ojemann, R. G., Nadol, J. B., Montgomery, W. W., Levine, R. A., Carlisle, E., & Martuza, R. (1992). Long-term hearing results in patients after surgical removal of acoustic tumors with hearing preservation. *The American Journal of Otology, 13* (2), 134–136.

Moller, A. (1987). Electrophysiological monitoring of cranial nerves in operations in the skull base. In Sekhar & Schramm (Eds.), *Tumors of the cranial base: Diagnosis and treatment* (pp. 123–132). Mount Kisco, NY: Futura Publishing Co.

Moller, A. (1992a). Physiology of the auditory system and recording of auditory evoked potentials. In J. Kartush & K. Bouchard (Eds.), *Neuromonitoring in otology and head and neck surgery* (pp. 163–198). New York: Raven Press.

Moller, A. (1992b). Use of brainstem auditory evoked potentials in intraoperative neurophysiologic monitoring. In J. Kartush & K. Bouchard (Eds.), *Neuromonitoring in otology and head and neck surgery* (pp. 199–214). New York: Raven Press.

Mustain, W. D., Al-Mefty, O., & Anand, V. K. (1992) Inconsistencies in the correlation between loss of brain stem auditory evoked response waves and postoperative deafness. *Journal of Clinical Monitoring, 8* (3), 231–235.

National Institutes of Health (NIH). (1991). Acoustic Neuroma. *Acoustic Neuroma Consensus Statement, 9* (4), 1–24.

Ruth, R. A., & Lambert, P. R. (1991). Auditory evoked potentials. *Clinical Audiology, Otolaryngologic Clinics of North America, 24* (2), 349–370.

Ruth, R. A., Lambert, P. R., & Ferraro, J. A. (1988). Electrocochleography: Methods and clinical applications. *The American Journal of Otology, 9* (Suppl.), 1–11.

Ruth, R. A., Mills, J. A., & Jane, J. A. (1986). Intraoperative monitoring of electrocochleographic and auditory brainstem responses. *Seminars in Hearing, 7* (3), 307–326.

Schwaber, M. K., Hall, J. W., & Zealer, D. L. (1991). Intraoperative monitoring of the facial and cochleovestibular nerves in otologic surgery: Part two. *Insights in Otolaryngology, 6* (6), 1–8.

Selters, W. (1993). ABR screening for acoustic tumors. *Seminars in Hearing, 14* (2), 134–142.

Shelton, C., Brackmann, D. E., House, W. F., & Hitselberger, W. E. (1989). Acoustic tumor surgery: Prognostic factors in hearing conservation. *Archives of Otolaryngolology—Head and Neck Surgery, 115,* 1213–1216.

Shelton, C., Hitselberger, W. E., House, W. F., & Brackmann, D. E. (1990). Hearing preservation after acoustic tumor removal: Long term results. *Laryngoscope, 100,* 115–119.

Sininger, Y. S., & Masuda, A. (1990). Effect of click polarity on ABR threshold. *Ear and Hearing, 11* (3), 206–209.

Starr, A., McPherson, D., Patterson, J., Don, M., Luxford, W., Shannon, R., Sininger, Y., Tonokawa, L., & Waring, M. (1991). Absence of both auditory evoked potentials and auditory percepts dependent on timing cues. *Brain, 114,* 1157–1180.

Swan, I. R. C., & Browning, G. G. (1989). Imaging patients with suspected acoustic neuroma [Letter to the Editor]. *Lancet,* 219.

Telian, S. A., Kileny, P. R., Niparko, J. K., Kemink, J. L., & Graham, M. D. (1989). Normal auditory brainstem response in patients with acoustic neuroma. *Laryngoscope, 99,* 10–14.

von Glass, W., Haid, C., Cidlinsky, K., Stenglein, C., & Christ, P. (1991). False-positive MR imaging in the diagnosis of acoustic neurinomas. *Otolaryngology— Head and Neck Surgery, 104* (6), 863–866.

Welling, D. B., Glasscock, M. E., Woods, C. I., & Jackson, C. G. (1990). Acoustic neuroma: A cost-effective approach. *Otolaryngology—Head and Neck Surgery, 103* (3), 364–370.

Wilson, D. F., Hodgson, R. S., Gustafson, M. F., Hogue, S., & Mills, L. (1992). The sensitivity of auditory brainstem response testing in small acoustic neuromas. *Laryngoscope, 102,* 961–964.

■ CHAPTER 6 ■

MONITORING THE VAGUS NERVE

■ DOUGLAS L. BECK, M.A. ■
■ GARY R. LaBLANCE, Ph.D. ■

Postoperative vocal fold paralysis and paresis are complications associated with a variety of surgical procedures. The exact occurrence rate is unknown, as some of these injuries are transient and some are unreported. The procedures that appear to present the most risk for iatrogenic injury include thyroidectomy, parathyroidectomy, coronary artery bypass, carotid endarterectomy, and other procedures involving the upper torso and neck. Postoperative hoarseness is often ascribed to extubation. Inadvertent and unrecognized manipulation of the recurrent laryngeal nerve (RLN) is probably partially responsible for these injuries.

ANATOMY

The vagus nerve emerges in the midbrain from the nucleus ambiguus of the medulla oblongata, between the cerebellar peduncle and the inferior olives (Figure 6–1). The nerve exits the skull through the jugular foramen and divides into many branches that serve the head, neck, thorax, and abdomen.

Immediately after exiting the skull, several nerve branches leave the vagus and join with other cranial nerves to supply sensory fibers to the head.

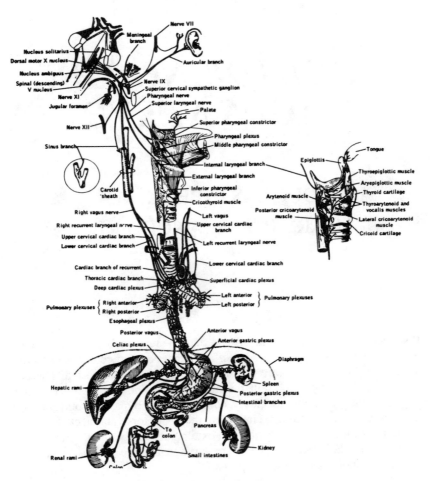

FIGURE 6–1. The vagus nerve anatomy. (From *A Functional Approach in Neuroanatomy*. By E. House and B. Pansky, 1967, New York: McGraw-Hill. Copyright 1967 by McGraw-Hill Book Company. Reprinted by permission.)

One of these branches, the meningeal filament, serves the dura mater on the posterior fossa of the base of the skull. A second branch, the auricular nerve branch, innervates the integument of the posterior portion of the external auditory meatus. A third branch, the pharyngeal nerve, supplies the majority of the muscles and mucous membrane of the pharynx and soft palate.

The major portions of the vagus serving the larynx are the superior laryngeal and the recurrent laryngeal nerves. The superior laryngeal nerve arises from the inferior ganglion and descends along the pharynx. Immediately below the inferior ganglion, it divides into two branches, the internal and external laryngeal nerves.

The internal laryngeal nerve descends to enter the larynx through the thyrohyoid membrane, where it further divides into the upper and lower branches. The internal laryngeal nerve contains afferent fibers from the mucosa in the ipsilateral supraglottis and from the base of the tongue. It also contains fibers from muscle spindles and other stretch receptors in the larynx. The external laryngeal nerve is an efferent branch of the superior laryngeal nerve that descends posteriorly to the sternothyroid muscle and innervates the cricothyroid muscle and the inferior pharyngeal constrictor.

The remaining laryngeal musculature is supplied by the recurrent laryngeal nerve. This nerve pair, unlike the rest that supply the larynx, is not bilaterally symmetric. The left recurrent laryngeal nerve descends into the thorax where it exits the vagal trunk, loops around the aortic arch, and then ascends in the tracheoesophageal groove to enter the larynx through the cricothyroid membrane. The right recurrent laryngeal nerve exits the vagal trunk at the level of the subclavian artery and then passes under it and the right common carotid artery before ascending to enter the larynx. The nerve on both sides divides into an anterior and posterior branch. The anterior branch supplies the lateral cricoarytenoid and thyroarytenoid muscles. The posterior branch supplies the posterior cricoarytenoid and the interarytenoid muscles. The mucosa of the infraglottis receives afferent information from the recurrent laryngeal nerve (RLN).

As the vagus continues to descend, small branches exit the main trunk to supply many structures in the thorax and abdomen. The superior and inferior cardiac nerve branches of the vagus serve the cardiac plexus, while the anterior and posterior bronchial branches provide sensory fibers to the lungs and the esophageal branch supplies afferent fibers to the esophagus. In the abdomen, the gastric branch supplies sensory fibers to the stomach; the celiac branch supplies sensory fibers to the pancreas, spleen, kidneys, and the intestines; and the hepatic branch provides sensory fibers to the liver.

HISTORICAL REVIEW

The contemporary methods employed to monitor the RLN during surgery continue to develop. A cursory review of the basic monitoring systems demonstrates a need for further development and refinement. The common problem with most "needle based" RLN monitoring systems is confirmation of and access to the recording electrode insertion site.

Although one can easily determine that the electrodes are intact, the impedances are acceptable, and the recording system is properly operating, confirmation of the recording electrode position within the target tissue can only be accomplished using direct visual observation.

Beck and Maves (1992) report on two monitoring techniques. The first was used with patients who presented with large thyroids. Teflon-coated silver wires in a bipolar hookwire configuration (Figure 6–2) were placed in the vocalis muscle after intubation but before the start of the surgical procedure. Although these electrodes are very sensitive and highly specific, they were difficult to insert using an intraoral approach. Nonetheless, this was accomplished by the surgeon using direct visualization through a laryngoscope.

The second technique was used with patients presenting with smaller thyroids. This technique used standard subdermal monopolar needle electrodes placed in the vocalis muscle following minimal surgical exposure. Thus, visualization of the insertion site was easily accomplished. This technique is lacking in that iatrogenic injury may occur before the electrodes are in place, allowing potentially "false negative" responses to occur.

Lipton, McCaffrey, and Litchy (1988) describe a technique incorporating bipolar hookwire recording electrodes and an endoscopic visualization to verify proper in situ placement.

Woltering, Dumond, Ferrara, Farrar, and James (1984) present a monitoring technique involving a double-cuffed endotracheal tube. Their method allows standard intubation, inflates with low pressure, and monitors vocal fold motion secondary to recurrent laryngeal nerve stimulation via the detection of pressure changes within the expansion chamber.

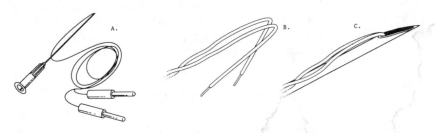

FIGURE 6–2. Bipolar hookwire electrodes in various stages of preparation: **A.** Teflon-coated silver wire placed within the 22-gauge needle. **B.** Demonstration of bare ends of silver following Teflon removal. **C.** Close-up view showing wires inserted into the needle tip.

Gavilan and Gavilan (1986) report an easy, low cost, basic method to monitor the RLN. The authors describe intraoperative placement of the surgeon's fingers within the larynx to verify motoric motion while electrically stimulating the RLN with a disposable stimulator.

RECENT DEVELOPMENTS

Perhaps as a follow-up to the Woltering et al. (1984) technique noted above, a modified endotracheal tube is now manufactured by Xomed Treace (Figure 6–3). This endotracheal tube features bipolar stainless steel wires on the exterior of the tube. The steel wires contact the vocal folds, allowing recordings of EMG activity based on vocal fold motion.

THE GOAL

As is true with all intraoperative monitoring, the goal is to avoid iatrogenic injury. This is accomplished primarily by using an "early warning system" sensitive enough to warn the surgical team of a potential problem before it becomes a permanent injury. Prevention of postoperative vocal fold paresis and paralysis may be efficiently accomplished by monitoring the EMG response from the RLN.

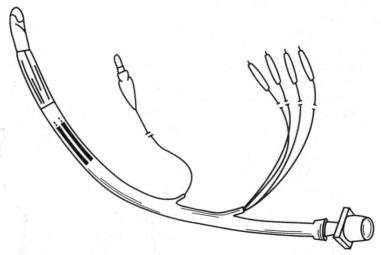

FIGURE 6–3. Xomed-Treace RLN monitoring endotracheal tube. (Used with permission of Xomed-Treace, Jacksonville, Florida.)

ANESTHESIA

As the monitored structure (RLN) is a motor nerve, and because the published data are currently nondefinitive regarding stimulation levels and related concerns, it is best not to use neuromuscular blockade following intubation. This is a decision that needs to be addressed by the surgeon and the anesthesiologist.

RECORDING ELECTRODE PLACEMENT

Intraoperative monitoring of the vagus nerve may be performed with concentric needles, subdermal needles, hookwire electrodes, or the endotracheal intubation tube protocol such as that manufactured by Xomed-Treace, Inc.

Bipolar hookwire electrodes use a hypodermic needle as a "carrier" to achieve proper placement in a muscle group. The wire(s) may be silver, platinum, or copper and are usually coated with Teflon. This type of electrode is most useful for evaluating the larynx during dynamic activities and long-term monitoring (Lovelace, Blitzer, & Ludlow, 1992).

False-positive findings are greatly reduced with bipolar hookwire electrodes; these are very sensitive and eliminate most artifact (Beck & Maves, 1991). Electrodes may be placed in the thyroarytenoid muscle using either a percutaneous or intraoral route.

Percutaneous placements are achieved by positioning the electrode in the midline of the larynx and advancing it through the epithelium and the cricothyroid membrane. Once the membrane is pierced, the needle is directed superiorly and laterally until it enters the muscle. An anterior angle of insertion is preferred; electrodes that are positioned too far posteriorly are more likely to enter the lateral cricoarytenoid muscle. According to Schaefer (1991), percutaneous recordings may be made with either multipolar concentric or bipolar hookwire electrodes. Intraoral insertions are made either by direct laryngoscopy or by electrode insertion forceps guided by fiberoptic laryngoscopy (Thumfart, 1988).

Placement of electrodes into the posterior cricoarytenoid muscle may also be accomplished by either a percutaneous or an intraoral route. A percutaneous placement can be performed when minimal subcutaneous neck fat is present.

In these cases, the anterior larynx is rotated away from the recording site to allow greater access to the posterior aspect of the cricoid cartilage. The electrode is passed immediately posterior to the thyroid lamina at the level of the superior half of the cricoid cartilage until it reaches the rostrum.

In intraoral insertions, the electrode is passed into the pharynx and subsequently into the larynx while monitoring needle placement via direct or fiberoptic laryngoscopy. Forceps may be used to assist recording electrode placement.

The cricothyroid muscle can be monitored through a percutaneous placement of the electrode. The needle is inserted through the midline epithelium superior to the cricoid prominence and is advanced superiorly and laterally along the cricoid cartilage until the cricothyroid muscle is pierced. Recordings from the sternohyoid, sternothyroid, and sternomastoid muscles may be excluded when no motor unit potentials are achieved during movements of the head. An intraoral approach cannot be used effectively to reach the cricothyroid muscle (Lovelace et al., 1992).

STIMULATION FACTORS

Stimulating electrodes may be monopolar or bipolar. The monopolar electrodes have a single-prong design. The cathode is hand-held and the anode is outside the surgical field. The flexibility of this design allows stimulation if visualization of the anatomy is difficult or impossible.

Bipolar stimulating electrodes have a two-prong design; the distance between the cathode and anode may be variable or fixed. The benefit of bipolar stimulation is that the stimulation area is restricted. The majority of electrical excitation occurs between the two prongs, minimizing false-positives.

Although no firm guidelines exist for stimulation levels, conservative levels are clearly preferred. Using a constant current stimulator, current can be delivered at 0.20 mA, and slowly raised until a repeatable, well-defined contraction occurs. Excessive stimulation may result in a transient paralysis.

FUTURE DIRECTIONS

Electromyographic (EMG) observations are dependent on the recording technique, the type and placement of the recording electrodes, and the stimulation protocols. Quantification of laryngeal EMG is difficult because muscles act as an electrical filter and may diminish high-frequency activity or may pass low-frequency artifact. In addition, many factors influence the pattern of the action potentials. Patient age, muscle bulk, and body temperature influence the motor unit potentials.

Future research should focus on hardware and software systems designed to improve the sensitivity of the recording systems and reduce artifact. Placement problems need to be thoroughly investigated to enhance the percutaneous and intraoral methods of insertion. The efficacy of systems that combine simultaneous video fiberoptic monitoring and electromyographic assessment should be carefully examined.

REFERENCES

Beck, D., & Maves, M. (1991). Intraoperative monitoring during parotid and thyroid surgery using the nerve integrity monitor-2. An application note for Xomed Treace Mfg. Co., Jacksonville, FL.

Beck, D., & Maves, M. (1992). Recurrent laryngeal nerve monitoring. In J. M. Kartush & K. R. Bouchard (Eds.), *Neuromonitoring in otology and head and neck surgery*, (pp. 151-162). New York: Raven Press.

Gavilan, J., & Gavilan, C. (1986). Recurrent laryngeal nerve: Identification during thyroid and parathyroid surgery. *Archives of Otolaryngology Head Neck Surgery, 112*, 1286-1288.

Lipton, R. J., McCaffrey, T. V., & Litchy, W. J. (1988). Intraoperative electrophysiologic monitoring of laryngeal muscle during thyroid surgery. *Laryngoscope, 98*, 1292.

Lovelace, R. E., Blitzer, A., & Ludlow, C. L. (1992). Clinical laryngeal electromyography. In A. Blitzer, M. F. Brin, C. T. Sasaki, S. Fahn, & K. S. Harris (Eds.), *Neurologic disorders of the larynx* (pp. 66-81). New York: Thieme Medical Publishers.

Schaefer, S. D. (1991). Laryngeal electromyography. In J.A. Koufman & G. Isaacson (Eds.), *The otolaryngologic clinics of North America* (pp. 1053-1059). Philadelphia: W.B. Saunders Company.

Thumfart, W. F. (1988). Electrodiagnosis of laryngeal nerve disorders. *Ear, Nose, Throat Journal, 67*, 380-393.

Woltering, E. A., Dumond, D., Ferrara, J., Farrar, W. B., & James, A. G. (1984). A method for intraoperative identification of the recurrent laryngeal nerve. *The American Journal of Surgery, 148*, 438-440.

■ CHAPTER 7 ■

MONITORING THE SPINAL ACCESSORY NERVE

■ JOANNE M. SLATER, M.S. ■
■ DOUGLAS L. BECK, M.A. ■
■ KAREN YAFFEE, M.D. ■

ANATOMY AND PHYSIOLOGY

The spinal accessory nerve (SAN), CN XI, is primarily a motor nerve innervating the ipsilateral sternocleidomastoid (SCM) and trapezius muscles. It consists of cranial and spinal portions. The cranial fibers originate in the caudal portion of the nucleus ambiguus and run laterally toward the jugular foramen. The spinal portion arises from the motor cells of the anterior column of the gray matter from the upper five cervical nerve rootlets (Hollinshead, 1982). These rootlets emerge posteriorly and extend rostrally through the foramen magnum to enter the posterior cranial fossa and course toward the jugular foramen. At the jugular foramen is an interchange of filaments from the spinal and cranial portions of the SAN. In addition, fibers from the vagus nerve become intertwined (Brandenburg & Lee, 1981; Lanser, Jackler, & Yingling 1992). See Figure 7-1.

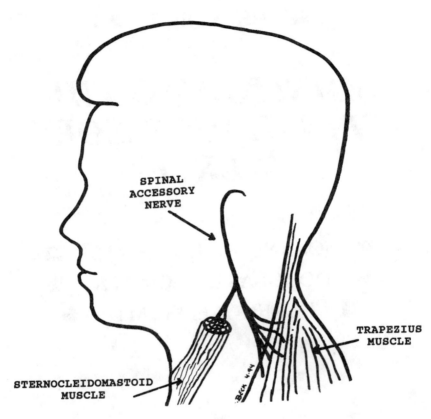

FIGURE 7–1. Basic anatomy of the spinal accessory nerve.

Below the level of the jugular foramen, the nerve courses behind the digastric and stylohyoid muscles and laterally to the internal jugular vein. It then runs obliquely downward to reach the medial surface of the SCM at the junction between its superior one-third and inferior two-thirds border. The nerve proceeds beneath the SCM and appears at its posterior border near the greater auricular nerve (Erb's point). The SAN then runs through the posterior triangle beneath the superficial layer of the deep cervical fascia to cross the anterior border of the trapezius approximately 2–3 cm above the clavicle (Lingeman, 1993).

Injury to the SAN may result in several unpleasant and disabling sequellae believed to be associated with denervation of the trapezius. These have been described as a syndrome including nonlocalized shoulder pain, limited abduction of the shoulder above 90° with a full passive range of motion, winging of the scapula, drooping shoulder, and an abnormal electromyogram of the trapezius muscle (Nahum, Mullally, & Marmor, 1961). Patients who sustain injury to the SAN report difficulty performing everyday tasks that require elevation of the arm on the involved side such as combing their hair, reaching for items on shelves, or removing a sweater (Short, Kaplan, Laramore, & Cummings, 1984; Sweeney & Wilbourn, 1992).

NECK DISSECTIONS

There are several surgical procedures that compromise the SAN. Neck dissections are the most frequent cause of iatrogenic injury to the SAN. Procedures in the vicinity of the cervical spine, posterior cranial fossa, jugular foramen, and the foramen magnum may also pose a threat to the SAN (Lanser et al., 1992). SAN injury is a rare complication of carotid endarterectomies (Maniglia & Han, 1991; Sweeney & Wilbourn, 1992; Tucker, Gee, Nicholas, McDonald, & Goodreau, 1987).

Iatrogenic injury to the SAN resulting from neck dissection has long been a source of discussion and controversy. The decision to perform radical versus modified neck dissection requires the surgeon to balance oncological safety and postoperative morbidity. Clearly, the SAN should only be preserved if there is no indication of metastasis to the nodes intimately related to the nerve. However, the specific factors weighed in the decision to perform a modified neck dissection are beyond the scope of this chapter.

A modified neck dissection can be defined as any technique that spares structures such as the SAN, the internal jugular vein, or the SCM (Medina, 1993). Postoperative comparisons of radical neck dissection versus this structure-sparing surgery (modified neck dissection) reveal variable results.

Generally, there are fewer complications following a modified neck dissection. Patients report a lower incidence or less severe symptoms of shoulder pain and less subjective difficulty performing daily tasks. There are fewer physical signs of trapezius dysfunction such as muscle atrophy, drooping of the shoulder, or scapular winging. Electromyography, range of motion testing, and tests of muscle strength reveal better functional performance of the trapezius (Leipzig, Suen, English, Barnes, & Hooper, 1983; Saunders, Hirata, & Jacques, 1985; Short, Kaplan, Laramore, & Cummings, 1984; Sobol, Jensen, Sawyer, Costiloe, & Thong, 1985; Zibordi, Baiocco, Bascelli, Bini, & Canepa, 1988).

Occasional complaints of shoulder pain and dysfunction persist follow-ing modified neck dissections in which the SAN was thought to have been preserved (Saunders et al., 1985; Short et al., 1984; Zibordi et al., 1988). Such problems have been attributed to stretching or devascularizing the nerve by manipulation at the time of surgery. Although surgical expertise certainly contributes to successful outcome, variability in postoperative results (by a single surgical group) suggests that shoulder function is influenced by several factors difficult to control and assess (DeSanto & Beahrs, 1988; Eisele & Weymuller, 1991).

In 1943, Seddon classified nerve injuries into three categories. The first is *neuropraxia*, a temporary blockage of nerve impulse conduction without structural damage. Once the blockage is removed, the nerve fibers recover. The second type of injury is *axonotmesis*, in which the neuron sheath remains intact, but the axon is disrupted. Orderly regeneration of the axon is supported by the continuous conduit provided by the sheath. Finally, *neurotmesis* in-volves complete transection of the nerve. In this case, orderly regeneration of the nerve fibers is nearly impossible (Seddon, 1943).

Variability in postoperative results may possibly be explained by the type of nerve injury sustained. A complete iatrogenic transection of the nerve may be obvious to the surgeon at the moment of injury. However, other injuries sustained by the nerve (e.g., "stretch injuries" and tearing of neural fibers with traction) may not be apparent without intraoperative monitoring of the SAN (Beck & Maves, 1991a, 1991b).

INTRAOPERATIVE MONITORING OF THE SAN

As with other motor nerves, intraoperative monitoring of the SAN is accomp-lished by inserting electrodes into the innervated musculature and transmit-ting auditory and visual information to the operator. Neural discharges from mechanical manipulation of the nerve, thermal changes, or electrical stimu-lation cause muscle contractions that are manifested as "real time" changes in EMG. These changes may be communicated to the surgeon verbally by the personnel operating the monitor or broadcast acoustically by the monitoring equipment. Monitoring provides instantaneous acoustic feedback to the surgeon about the status of the nerve.

ELECTRODES

Electrode placement for SAN monitoring is shown in Figure 7–2. After the patient is intubated and the skin is prepared with alcohol, bipolar hookwire electrodes are inserted into the sternocleidomastoid and trapezius muscles. A

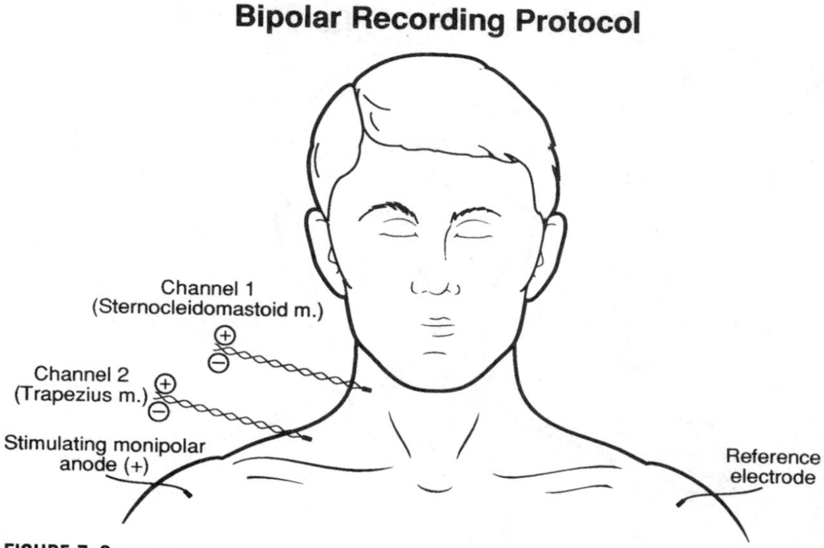

Bipolar Recording Protocol

FIGURE 7–2. Bipolar recording profile.

monopolar subdermal needle electrode is placed as a reference in the opposite shoulder. The stimulating anode, also a monopolar needle electrode, is placed in the ipsilateral deltoid muscle. Impromptu disturbance of the electrodes may be avoided by securing them with tape.

Bipolar hookwire electrodes are preferred for their specificity in monitoring responses of the muscles of interest. For a thorough description of their construction, the reader is referred to other sources (Beck & Benecke, 1990; Beck & Maves, 1991a). In essence, the last 1 mm of two strands of Teflon-coated silver wire are stripped of their insulation. The two exposed ends are inserted into the muscle via a needle. Only electrical activity occurring between these bare ends is identified as electromyography (EMG) by the monitoring equipment.

Monopolar electrodes have also been used successfully for recording purposes. (See Figure 7–3.) Pairs of subdermal needle electrodes are inserted into the musculature, set parallel and close to each other to achieve adequate response specificity (Kartush, Graham, & Bouchard, undated; Lanser et al., 1992).

ANESTHESIA

As stated in other chapters of this text and as is true with all motor nerve monitoring, the use of muscle relaxants postintubation is not desirable. The

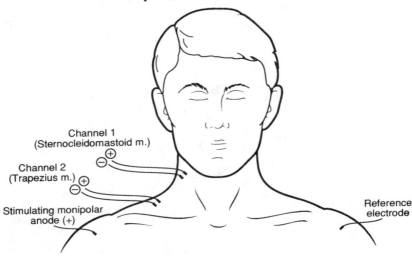

Monopolar Recording Protocol

Channel 1
(Sternocleidomastoid m.)

Channel 2
(Trapezius m.)

Stimulating monipolar
anode (+)

Reference
electrode

FIGURE 7–3. Monopolar recording profile.

monitoring personnel and the surgeon must consult with the anesthesia personnel on this important issue before the onset of general anesthesia.

Although low levels of neuromuscular blockade may be acceptable (allowing adequate EMG) while monitoring the SAN, the exact acceptable level is not known. Unfortunately, a low-level neuromuscular blockade may eliminate the opportunity to discover small, early changes in the EMG that might alert the surgeon to danger if the blockade were not administered.

EQUIPMENT

There are several commercially available systems for intraoperative cranial nerve monitoring. Their basic features should include an oscilloscope for visual display of ongoing EMG, an auditory monitor, and an electric nerve stimulator.

The Xomed-Treace Nerve Integrity Monitor-2 (NIM-2) is a battery-operated system used in the authors' practice. Use of a direct current power source isolates the NIM-2 from other power sources in the operating room, reducing electrical interference from other equipment. In addition, the NIM-2 offers flexibility in selection of stimulus parameters (such as rate, duration, and maximum output) and visual display parameters (such as the time scale and vertical display scale).

Simultaneous monitoring of CN IX through CN XII has been advocated by some authors for surgery of the posterior cranial fossa, jugular foramen,

foramen magnum, parapharyngeal space, and thyroid region (Lanser et al., 1992). Equipment requirements, although essentially the same, must accommodate monitoring of multiple cranial nerves. Such a system might employ a multichannel oscilloscope and allow for adjustment of individual amplifier characteristics. Electrodes may be placed solely in the trapezius muscle for SAN monitoring in such involved cases.

NERVE STIMULATION

The nerve stimulator may be utilized to map the location of the nerve in difficult anatomy prior to dissection. Either bipolar or monopolar stimulation can be used successfully, depending on the experience and the preference of the surgeon. A constant current stimulus from 0.20 to 1 mA is typically adequate to produce a response with a healthy nerve. Because very little is known regarding the effect of high amplitude electrical stimulation of cranial nerves, it is recommended that the lowest level that consistently yields a repeatable response be used.

MONITORED RESPONSE

The type and pattern of electrical activity monitored at the trapezius varies depending on its cause. Baseline EMG activity is shown in Figure 7–4A. Activity produced by electrical stimulation follows a rhythmic pattern of pulses that is time-locked to the stimulus. These pulses appear as spikes on the visual display and are heard as "beats" occurring at the same rate as the stimulus. (See Figure 7–4C.)

Generally, there is a relationship between the amplitude of the stimulus and the amplitude of the response (in microvolts) in a healthy nerve. This relationship may bear prognostic information regarding the SAN and trapezius function. Comparisons of facial nerve responses to electrical stimulation during surgery and postoperative facial motion have demonstrated that this

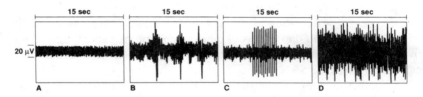

FIGURE 7–4. Representative EMG displays. **A.** Baseline EMG. **B.** Bursts of EMG from mechanical stimuli. **C.** Response to electrical stimulation. **D.** Neural traction.

essentially holds true for the facial nerve (Beck, Atkins, Benecke, & Brackmann, 1991). There are no reports of similar studies involving the SAN.

Mechanical stimuli also cause characteristic EMG patterns (Kartush et al., undated; Kartush & Prass, 1988). Brief mechanical contact with the nerve or musculature produces a single, audible "burst" of activity (see Figure 7–4B). The "tap test" takes advantage of this phenomenon. Prior to surgery, it is important to verify the integrity of the electrodes, their placement, and the monitoring equipment. If tapping on the musculature produces the expected visual and acoustic correlates of the muscle activity, it can be assumed that the equipment is properly installed for accurate monitoring. Mechanically evoked EMG during dissection may alert the surgeon to the proximity of the SAN before it can be visually identified. Activity associated with mechanical or electrical stimulation occurs immediately following the stimulus, allowing establishment of cause–effect relationships.

Certain surgical maneuvers, such as traction or stretching on the nerve, may produce repetitive neural firings, which are observed as continuous "trains" of electrical activity or an increase in the baseline activity (see Figure 7–4D). The resulting EMG may occur after the irritating surgical event (Kartush et al., undated).

Despite the relationship between different types of electrical activity and their frequently associated causes, the specific cause should not be determined merely by the type of activity observed. EMG activity must be interpreted in the surgical context in which it occurs. Familiarity with the anatomy and the procedure to be performed will optimize the benefit gained by intraoperative monitoring.

CONCLUSION

As electrophysiologic technology advances, the standard of patient care advances. The criteria for successful neck dissection previously consisted of tumor removal without patient mortality or recurrence of disease. Injury to the SAN, although a serious complication, was a secondary consideration compared to the patient's overall health.

However, preservation of the SAN is becoming increasingly possible with no added risk to the successful management of the patient. Intraoperative monitoring has provided an avenue for improvement of procedures that can compromise the SAN.

Whether or not to make the effort to spare the SAN is no longer the question. Efforts are now aimed at discerning how this is best accomplished. The application of intraoperative monitoring to procedures involving the SAN is not yet widespread, but may be a new avenue for intraoperative monitoring.

REFERENCES

Beck, D. L., Atkins, J. S., Benecke, J. E., & Brackmann, D. E. (1991). Intraoperative monitoring: Prognostic aspects during acoustic tumor removal. *Otolaryngology— Head and Neck Surgery, 106,* 780-782.

Beck, D. L., & Benecke, J. E. (1990). Intraoperative facial nerve monitoring technical aspects. *Otolaryngology—Head and Neck Surgery, 102,* 270-273.

Beck, D. L., & Maves, M. D. (1991a). Intraoperative monitoring during parotid and thyroid surgery using the Nerve Integrity Monitor-2. *Xomed-Treace Application Note.*

Beck, D. L., & Maves, M. D. (1991b). Spinal accessory nerve preservation. *Laryngoscope, 101,* 1386.

Brandenburg, J. H., & Lee, C. Y. (1981). The eleventh nerve in radical neck surgery. *Laryngoscope, 91,* 1851-1859.

DeSanto, L. W., & Beahrs, O. H. (1988). Modified and complete neck dissection in the treatment of squamous cell carcinoma of the head and neck. *Surgery, Gynecology and Obstetrics, 167,* 259-269.

Eisele, D. W., Weymuller, E. A., & Price, J. C. (1991). Spinal accessory nerve preservation during neck dissection. *Laryngoscope, 101,* 433-435.

Hollinshead, W. H. (1982). *Anatomy of the head and neck.* Philadelphia: Harper & Row.

Kartush, J. M., Graham, M. D., & Bouchard, K. R. (Undated). Intraoperative facial nerve monitoring at Michigan Ear Institute. *Xomed-Treace Application Note.*

Kartush, J. M., & Prass, R. L. (1988). *Facial nerve testing: Electroneurography and intraoperative monitoring.* Instruction Course presented at the annual convention of the American Academy of Otolaryngology—Head and Neck Surgery, San Diego.

Lanser, M., Jackler, R., & Yingling, C. (1992). Regional monitoring of the lower (ninth through twelfth) cranial nerves. In J. Kartush & K. Bouchard (Eds.), *Monitoring in otology and head and neck surgery* (pp. 131-150). New York: Raven Press.

Leipzig, B., Suen, J. Y., English, J. L., Barnes, J., & Hooper, M. (1983). Functional evaluation of the spinal accessory nerve after neck dissection. *The American Journal of Surgery, 146,* 526-530.

Lingeman, R. (1993). Surgical Anatomy. In C. Cummings (Ed.), *Otolaryngology— Head and neck surgery* (pp. 1530-1543). St. Louis: C. V. Mosby.

Maniglia, A. J., & Han, D. P. (1991). Cranial nerve injuries following carotid endarterectomy: An analysis of 336 procedures. *Head & Neck, 13,* 121-124.

Medina, J. E. (1993). Neck dissection. In C. Cummings (Ed.), *Otolaryngology—Head and neck surgery* (pp. 1649-1672). St. Louis: C. V. Mosby.

Nahum, A. M., Mullally, W., & Marmor, L. (1961). A syndrome resulting from radical neck dissection. *Archives of Otolaryngology, 74,* 424-428.

Saunders, J. R., Hirata, R. M., & Jacques, D. A. (1985). Considering the spinal accessory nerve in head and neck surgery. *The American Journal of Surgery, 155,* 491-494.

Seddon, H. J. (1943). Three types of nerve injury. *Brain,* 66, Part 4, 238–283.

Short, S. O., Kaplan, J. N., Laramore, G. E., & Cummings, C. W. (1984). Shoulder pain and function after neck dissection with or without preservation of the spinal accessory nerve. *The American Journal of Surgery, 148,* 478–482.

Sobol, S., Jensen, C., Sawyer, W., Costiloe, P., & Thong, N. (1985). Objective comparison of physical dysfunction after neck dissection. *The American Journal of Surgery, 150,* 503–509.

Sweeney, P. J., & Wilbourn, A. J. (1992). Spinal accessory (11th) nerve palsy following carotid endarterectomy. *Neurology, 42,* 674–675.

Tucker, J. A., Gee, W., Nicholas, G. G., McDonald, K. M., & Goodreau, J. J. (1987). Accessory nerve injury during carotid endarterectomy. *Journal of Vascular Surgery, 5,* 440–444.

Zibordi, F., Baiocco, F., Bascelli, C., Bini, A., & Canepa, A. (1988). Spinal accessory nerve function following neck dissection. *Annals of Otology, Rhinology, and Laryngology, 97,* 83–86.

■ CHAPTER 8 ■

MONITORING THE HYPOGLOSSAL NERVE

■ AUKSE E. BANKAITIS, M.A. ■
■ ROBERT W. KEITH, Ph.D. ■

Intraoperative monitoring of the hypoglossal nerve (CN XII) is a logical and valuable extension of facial nerve (CN VII) monitoring (Moller, 1988). Because of the nature of various posterior fossa surgical procedures, we typically monitor CN XII in conjunction with multiple cranial nerves as well as the auditory brainstem response (ABR) and somatosensory cortical evoked potentials (SCEP). Determining when to monitor the hypoglossal nerve depends largely on the preoperative diagnosis, surgical procedure, and knowledge of pertinent anatomy. Familiarization with the anatomy of the hypoglossal nerve is a necessary building block for appreciating at what point the nerve may be at-risk.

BRAINSTEM ORIENTATION OF THE HYPOGLOSSAL NUCLEUS

There are 12 pairs of cranial nerves, each denoted by a Roman numeral corresponding to its emergence from the brainstem. Moving in a rostral-caudal direction, the designated numerical value of the nerves increases, so CN I is located near the midbrain at the level of the diencephalon, with the hypoglossal nerve (CN XII) surfacing at the level of the medulla (Bankaitis & Keith, 1993). Unlike the spinal nerves, all of which contain both efferent and afferent fibers, individual cranial nerves contain either motor only, sensory only, or sensory and motor (mixed) fibers. Of the 12 pairs of cranial nerves, the three extraocular nerves (CN III, CN IV, and CN VI) and the hypoglossal nerve (CN XII) contain only motor fibers. The motor nuclei of these four individual cranial nerve pairs form a vertical column along either side of the dorsal aspect of the brainstem midline with the oculomotor (CN III) and trochlear (CN IV) nuclei respectively, located at the level of the rostral and caudal midbrain, the abducens (CN VI) nucleus situated within the pons, and nucleus of the hypoglossal nerve (CN XII) located at the level of the medulla.

ANATOMY OF THE HYPOGLOSSAL NERVE

The hypoglossal nerve (CN XII) originates from the ipsilateral hypoglossal nucleus located in the tegmentum of the medulla. This motor nucleus forms a triangular shaped protrusion in the floor of the fourth ventricle known as the hypoglossal trigone. From its nucleus, the hypoglossal nerve courses ventrally to emerge as a series of rootlets in a groove between the medullary pyramids and the olive (Nolte, 1988). As the hypoglossal nerve exits the cranium by way of the hypoglossal foramen, it courses between the internal carotid artery and internal jugular vein (Zemlin, 1988). As it descends from its origin, the hypoglossal nerve courses lateral to the bifurcation of the common carotid artery and loops anteriorly above the great cornu of the hyoid bone (Wilson-Pauwels, Akesson, & Stewart, 1988). The motor fibers of the hypoglossal nerve distribute to supply all of the intrinsic muscles and most of the extrinsic muscles of the tongue.

LESIONS OF CRANIAL NERVE XII

Unilateral injuries of the hypoglossal nucleus or peripheral damage to the nerve fibers may result in paralysis and atrophy of the muscles of the ipsilateral half of the tongue. On protrusion, the tongue deviates toward the paralyzed side becuase of the unopposed contraction of the opposite genioglossus muscle (Zemlin, 1988). Movements of the protruded tongue toward the unaffected side are absent or weak. It is important to note that an upper motor neuron lesion affecting the musculature of the tongue will result in deviation of the tongue away from the side of the lesion (Zemlin, 1988). The hypoglossal nerve may, in rare instances, suffer a bilateral injury, causing impairment of lateral tongue mobility accompanied by atrophy on both sides of tongue (Kenrick, Bredfeldt, Sheridan, & Monroe, 1977).

The medial portion of medulla is supplied by a branch of the vertebral artery known as the anterior spinal artery. As the hypoglossal nucleus is located at the level of the medulla, infarction of the anterior spinal artery or the vertebral artery may damage the nucleus and/or fibers of the hypoglossal nerve. In addition, compression of the hypoglossal nerve by a tortuous internal carotid artery may result in complications (Scottig, Melancon, & Oliver, 1978). Other causes of hypoglossal nerve damage include late complications of radiation therapy of head and neck carcinoma, acute anterior poliomyelitis, infectious polyneuritis, neurofibromatosis, and syringomyelia (Cheng & Schultz (1975).

INTRAOPERATIVE MONITORING TECHNIQUE

The purpose of monitoring the hypoglossal nerve is to assist in early nerve identification during any surgical procedure that may jeopardize the postoperative functional integrity of the nerve (Kartush, 1989). We have monitored hypoglossal nerve function in patients with brainstem arterial venous malformation (AVM) and aneurysm, clival tumors, brainstem meningiomas, as well as for other patients for whom the lesion and, therefore, the operative procedure, involved the medulla, floor of the fourth ventricle, and foramen magnum.

EQUIPMENT

Although evoked potential equipment can be used to monitor cranial nerve function, most of the neurosurgical cases we monitor involve simultaneous, on-line monitoring of the ABR, SEP, and one or more cranial nerves. As a result, we prefer a multiple-channel electromyographic (EMG) recording system, such as the Nerve Integrity Monitor-2 (NIM-2, Xomed-Treace, Inc., Jacksonville, Florida; [Figure 8-1]). The visual and auditory feedback of EMG activity provided by the NIM-2 provides the intraoperative personnel with the flexibility to simultaneously monitor pertinent cranial nerves acoustically while visually diverting attention to the continuous collection and interpretation of the ABR and SEP waveforms. The NIM-2 also contains muting circuitry that eliminates the electrical artifact associated with the use of electrocautery equipment throughout the surgical procedure. It is impor-

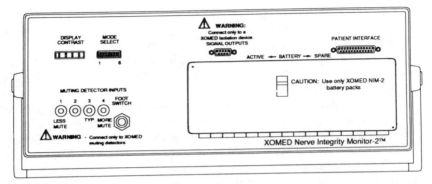

FIGURE 8-1. The Nerve Integrity Monitor-2 (NIM-2, Xomed-Treace, Inc., Jacksonville, Florida), a two-channel EMG recording system, is equipped with a dual feedback system. During neurosurgical cases that require on-line monitoring of various cranial nerves and evoked potentials, the NIM-2 provides not only visual feedback on a central screen, but auditory feedback via a speaker. Cranial nerves may be monitored acoustically while visual attention may be diverted to monitoring other potentials, such as the auditory brainstem response.

tant to keep in mind that valid monitoring of cranial nerves does not occur during electrocautery (Kartush & Bouchard, 1992); however, increase in background EMG activity immediately following the use of electrocautery equipment may be indicative of potential damage to the nerve.

ANESTHESIA

As discussed in our chapter on extraocular cranial nerve monitoring, anytime cranial nerve function is monitored, long-acting muscle relaxants or neuro-muscular blocking agents should be avoided. Even low doses of muscle relaxants that do not effect nerve responses from direct electrical stimulation may compromise the EMG. However, intraoperative monitoring often extends beyond cranial nerve monitoring to include concurrent monitoring of SEP. As most anesthetic agents significantly influence either the EMG or SEP resolution, anesthetic flexibility is often significantly restricted. For example, a deep anesthetic with volatile agents in an unparalyzed patient is optimum for cranial nerve EMG recordings; however, in situations in which brainstem function is simultaneously monitored, the amplitudes of upper SEP are significantly diminished (Hogan, 1992). Collaborative, not combative, communication between the anesthesiologist and neurophysiological intraoperative monitoring personnel prior to and throughout the surgical procedure is a necessary step toward providing quality intraoperative monitoring.

ELECTRODE POSITIONING

Once the patient is anesthetized, intubated, and positioned, a tongue depressor may be used to manipulate the oral cavity for positioning of electrodes. Two subdural needle electrodes are inserted into the anterior portion of the tongue on the operative side and the electrode leads are carefully taped to the face to maintain their position throughout the surgical procedure. Alternatively, a single electrode can be placed in the tongue with a reference subdermal electrode in the opposite forehead. Once electrode position is secured, the leads are connected to the patient interface box (Figure 8–2), and electrode impedances verified.

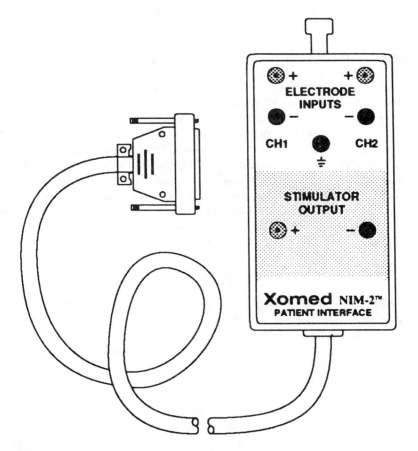

FIGURE 8-2. Needle electrode leads are inserted accordingly in the patient interface box which is connected to the back panel of the Nerve Integrity Monitor-2 (NIM-2, Xomed-Treace, Inc., Jacksonville, Florida).

As the test environment of the operating room contains multiple potential sources of electrical interference as well as limited access to the patient (Hall, 1992), obtaining the lowest possible electrode impedances (less than 5,000 ohms) is desirable because higher electrode impedances are more susceptible to the detection of electromagnetic noise (Prass, 1992).

STIMULATING PROBES

The stimulating probe is a hand-held device designed to deliver a specific amount of electrical current on direct contact with intracranial matter. Contact between the stimulating probe and intact nerve fibers will initiate the propagation of a nerve action potential toward the neuromuscular junction, producing contraction of intrinsic musculature of the tongue.

There are two types of stimulating probes available: monopolar and bipolar. Monopolar stimulation is suitable for mapping the general vicinity of the nerve, allowing for desired spread of current beyond the probe tip, with bipolar stimulation being much more selective, as it reduces the incidence of false-positive errors occurring from current spread (Kartush & Bouchard, 1992).

In the absence of established safety limitations for cranial nerve stimulation, we recommend the smallest amount of current stimulus necessary to elicit a detectable EMG event. Initially, we manually adjust the current stimulus at 0.05 mA; however, identification of cranial nerves in the presence of tumor mass may require higher levels of current stimulation. We increase current levels on request of the surgeon and strive to avoid stimulus levels exceeding 1 mA. Caution must be used when operating equipment capable of generating high current levels. The best guide is to use minimum stimulus current levels capable of producing a sufficient EMG response for monitoring.

INTERPRETATION OF RESPONSES

The EMG activity occurring during surgery may be described as nonrepetitive or repetitive. Nonrepetitive EMG activity exhibits a "burst" quality, with a typical duration of less than 1 sec and is most often associated with brief mechanical stimulation of the nerve(s) (Prass & Luders, 1986). Repetitive activity is typically associated with tumor extrapolation or compression of the nerve and nearby structures and may cease or decrease immediately following discontinuation of the surgical manipulation. Long duration increases of background EMG at any time during the surgical procedure may be indicative of potential damage to the nerve postoperatively.

In addition to mechanical stimulation, cranial nerve responses may occur as a result of other factors. Drilling adjacent to a nerve may transmit vibrations through surrounding bone, inducing what Kartush and Bouchard

(1992) refer to as a "drill potential." Thermal changes as a result of cold water irrigations and use of electrocautery equipment may evoke responses. Direct electrical stimulation of a functionally intact nerve produces synchronous responses or "pulses." However, reduction in the amplitude of an EMG response to direct stimulation indicates that the nerve is intact but there may be functional complications postoperatively. In addition, a nerve may be intact and functioning at the time of surgery, but postoperative edema may result in reduced functioning.In addition, preoperative and intraoperative communication with the surgical staff is extremely important—not only to confirm procedural expectations, but also to reduce unnecessary assumptions or confusion that may occur during the surgical procedure.

CASE STUDY

A 30-year-old-male diagnosed with a brainstem arterial venous malformation (AVM) was prepared for a suboccipital craniotomy and electrophysiological intraoperative monitoring for removal of the AVM. Electrophysiologic intraoperative monitoring of brainstem function was conducted using auditory brainstem responses and upper somatosensory cortical evoked potentials (SCEP). Insert earphones were placed in both ears, with SCEP stimulus needle electrode pairs inserted in the median nerve at each wrist. Response electrodes were appropriately placed at C3, C4, A1, A2 referenced to FZ.

Multiple cranial nerves were monitored with needle electrodes appropriately placed as:

Cranial Nerve		Electrode Placement
Trigeminal	(V)	Temporalis muscle
Abducens	(VI)	Rim of orbit at lateral canthus near lateral rectus muscle
Facial	(VII)	Orbicularis oris muscle
Vagus	(X)	Vocalis muscle
Accessory	(XI)	Trapezius muscle
Hypoglossal	(XII)	Tongue

To monitor the vagus nerve, we instructed anesthesiology to insert a single needle electrode into the lateral aspect of the vocalis muscle with a reference to the opposite forehead. Care must be taken in such placement to carefully tape the electrode lead to the patient's chin so as to remove any tension and reduce the chance of the electrode being dislodged during surgery.

When the dura was opened, attempts were made to identify cranial nerve pathways by stimulating the floor of the fourth ventricle. A stimulus intensity of 0.05 mA at 4 pulses per sec was utilized, with presentations through a Prass monopolar stimulus electrode. We were unable to identify absolutely the VI cranial nerves nuclei, because it was unclear if the response we obtained was from the lateral rectus or the nearby orbicularis oculi muscle. CN VII responded bilaterally, with responses of 1,600 μV. There was never any response from the vocalis muscle. CN XII was not stimulated.

We were able to obtain a response from the floor of the IV ventricle to CN XII with response amplitudes of 440 μV from the tongue. Following removal of the AVM, a response from CN VII nerve was identified on both the right and left sides of the response post AVM removal. The response amplitude was 130 μV representing a 90% reduction in response amplitude. In addition, CN XII nucleus was stimulated with a response amplitude of 120 μV representing a 70% reduction in response amplitude. The patient woke with normal cranial nerve function. This patient belies the notion that reduction of response amplitude will always result in paralysis. It may be that continued stimulation or irrigation and use of bipolar stimulation may immediately reduce nerve conduction, with relatively rapid recovery after closure. In addition, the patient represents a unique surgical situation, because responses were monitored from the floor of the fourth ventricle and not along the course of the nerve, as is normally done with facial nerve and other cranial nerve monitoring.

REFERENCES

Bankaitis, A., & Keith, R. (1993). Cranial nerve monitoring beyond the facial and auditory nerves. *Seminars in Hearing, 14* (2), 163–171.

Cheng, V., & Schultz M. (1975). Unilateral hypoglossal nerve atrophy as late complications of radiation therapy of head and neck carcinoma: A report of 4 cases and review of literature on peripheral and cranial nerve damages after radiation therapy. *Cancer, 35,* 1537–1544.

Hall, J. (1992). *Handbook of auditory evoked responses.* Boston: Allyn and Bacon.

Hogan, K. (1992). Neuroanesthetic techniques for intraoperative monitoring. In J. Kartush & K. Bouchard (Eds.), *Neuromonitoring in otology and head and neck surgery* (pp. 61–79). New York: Raven Press, Ltd.

Kartush, J., & Bouchard, K. (1992). Intraoperative facial nerve monitoring. In J. Kartush & K. Bouchard (Eds.), *Neuromonitoring in otology and head and neck surgery* (pp. 99–120). New York: Raven Press, Ltd.

Kartush, J. (1989). Electroneurography and intraoperative facial nerve monitoring in contemporary neurotology. *Otolaryngology—Head and Neck Surgery, 101,* 496–503.

Kenrick, M. Bredfeldt, R. Sheridan, C., & Monroe, A. (1977). Bilateral injury to the hypoglossal nerve. *Archives of Physical Medicine and Rehabilitation, 58,* 578–582.

Moller, A. (1988). *Evoked potentials in intraoperative monitoring.* Baltimore: Williams and Wilkins.

Nolte, J. (1988). *The human brain.* St. Louis: Mosby Year Book, Inc.

Prass, R. (1992). Intraoperative electromyographic recording. In J. Kartush & K. Bouchard (Eds.), *Neuromonitoring in otology and head and neck surgery* (pp. 81-98). New York: Raven Press, Ltd.

Prass, R., & Luders, H. (1986). Acoustic (loudspeaker) facial electromyographic monitoring: Part 1. *Neurosurgery, 19,* 392-400.

Scottig, D., Melancon, A., & Oliver, R. (1978). Hypoglossal paralysis due to compression by a tortuous internal carotid artery in the neck. *Neuroradiology, 14,* 263-265.

Wilson-Pauwels, L., Akesson, E., & Stewart, P. (1988). *Cranial nerves: Anatomy and clinical comments.* Toronto: B.C. Decker Inc.

Zemlin, W. (1988). *Speech and hearing science: Anatomy and physiology.* Englewood Cliffs, NJ: Prentice Hall.

■ SECTION TWO ■

SPINAL CORD MONITORING

CHAPTER 9

SOMATOSENSORY EVOKED POTENTIALS

■ ANNE M. PADBERG, M.S. ■

■ LESLIE S. HOLLAND, M.S. ■

In recent years, advances in technology and an expanse of clinical experience have led to the routine use of somatosensory evoked potentials (SEP) in the operating room. Evoked potentials are useful in determining the functional integrity of peripheral and central neural structures placed at-risk intraoperatively. SEP monitoring ideally serves as an early warning system to detect injury. SEPs may change the course of surgery and prevent irreversible damage (Bradshaw, Webb, & Fraser, 1984).

In these times of escalating health care costs, the efficacy of intraoperative monitoring is sometimes questioned. However, the cost is relatively insignificant when compared to the lifelong emotional and physical trauma and the financial expense incurred for the care of only one patient rendered paraplegic from an iatrogenic injury that could have possibly been detected with SEP monitoring and potentially reversed.

A thorough understanding of theory and applied technique is a prerequisite for anyone performing intraoperative SEP monitoring. The operating room is not an appropriate location for a beginner to start honing basic skills. It is strongly recommended, particularly for people working independently, that time be taken to become familiar with stimulation and recording of the SEP responses in an office/diagnostic setting. This type of experience will serve the beginner well in the operating room. The somatosensory evoked potential is elicited by stimulating either a sensory or mixed (sensory and motor) peripheral nerve. Stimulation is typically electrical (although mechanical or magnetic is possible) and of sufficient amplitude to elicit a response. Once elicited, the neural response can be recorded from various locations along the neural pathway. "Far field" recording techniques are employed and the response is displayed in waveforms of a distinct and recognizable pattern. (See Figure 9–1.)

The term "far field" refers to recording sites not in direct contact with neural structure producing activity. An example of this is using the surface of the skull to record a response from the brain. "Near field" recording means there is direct contact with the neural structure, such as placing electrodes on a peripheral nerve during surgery. Both methods are used intraoperatively for various types of surgical procedures.

SEP monitoring in an operative setting is performed to assess the functional status of peripheral nerves and sensory tracts in the spinal cord. Surgeries that require monitoring are those where the function of these structures are at-risk. This includes neurosurgical, orthopedic, and cardiothoracic cases. (See Table 9–1.)

ANESTHETIC CONSIDERATIONS FOR INTRAOPERATIVE SOMATOSENSORY EVOKED POTENTIAL MONITORING

Somatosensory evoked potentials in the operating room can be significantly affected by the anesthetic regimen. Cortical data are most sensitive to anesthesia, although to some extent all recorded responses may be affected. However, with a certain amount of cooperation from anesthesia personnel,

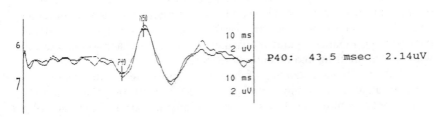

FIGURE 9–1. Typical cortical response measured following posterior tibial nerve stimulation.

TABLE 9–1. SURGICAL PROCEDURES GENERALLY MONITORED WITH SOMATOSENSORY EVOKED POTENTIALS.

Procedure	Etiology
Posterior spinal fusion with instrumentation	Idiopathic scoliosis Degenerative scoliosis Congenital scoliosis Neuromuscular disease Schuerman's kyphosis Spine fracture/trauma Metastatic carcinoma
Posterior decompression with or without instrumentation	Spinal stenosis Spondylolisthesis Herniated disc
Anterior spinal fusion with or without instrumentation	Fracture/trauma Scoliosis Degenerative disease Metastatic carcinoma
Carotid endarterectomy	Carotid artery disease
Aneurysm repair	Abdominal aortic aneurysm Cerebral aneurysm
Intra-extramedullary spinal cord surgery	Spinal cord tumor Metastatic carcinoma Arterial/venous malformation

reliable data can be obtained. Halogenated agents such as isoflurane or halothane are most often used in conjunction with nitrous oxide. These drugs have the most potential for reducing and sometimes obliterating cortical data. It is necessary to limit the amounts used to allow successful evoked potential monitoring. Typically, a concentration of 0.5% or less isoflurane or halothane and 50% or less nitrous oxide will allow reliable recording of data. Please keep in mind that this is not an absolute; some variance in either direction may be acceptable. Each patient may respond differently to anesthesia. However, this is an excellent guideline to use when faced with anesthetic protocol.

Narcotics usually provide a more favorable environment for recording evoked potential data. Suppression of cortical data is not as severe when they are used. There are two factors often encountered with narcotic anesthesia that may affect data. First, in the balanced anesthetic technique other drugs are frequently used in combination with a narcotic. These typically consist of nitrous oxide and/or halogenated agents. The same considerations have to be given regarding the amounts used. Fortunately, the use of narcotics in conjunction with other agents allows the anesthesiologist to use lower than usual doses of these other agents (for example, 0.25% isoflurane or 50% nitrous oxide). The second consideration is method of administration: continuous infusion or bolus injection. The continuous infusion method is preferable for evoked potential data. This method allows for maintenance of a relatively stable anesthetic plane. Bolus injection, which is a large dose given all at once, initially places a patient in a very deep level of anesthesia. This initial stage can preclude the recording of reliable data. The depth of anesthesia will gradually lessen and as this occurs, data will correspondingly improve. This continuous shifting of the anesthetic plane makes baseline data of little prognostic value and, if at all possible, should be avoided. This technique is most often encountered in cases of fairly short surgical duration. If there is no other option, it is important to be aware of when an injection is given and if it is repeated.

A narcotic deserving special attention is ketamine. Technically, this drug is a hypnotic but qualifies as an effective analgesic and amnesic. Ketamine has neuro excitatory properties that can enhance evoked potential data. In our operative setting, it is typically administered with a muscle relaxant and hypotensive agent. No other anesthetics are required with it and this further improves cortical evoked potential data (Nielsen, 1991).

Muscle relaxants are a routine part of most cases requiring evoked potential monitoring. They do not adversely affect responses, cortically or subcortically. It is necessary that a patient be relaxed to obtain relatively quiet data. Without muscle relaxants, subcortical data may become very noisy and contaminated with muscle artifact. The patient may also move when stimulated, if not adequately relaxed and this can obviously interfere with surgical procedures.

Other types of drugs are often used along with the previously discussed anesthetic regimens. Surgeries involving the spine or spinal cord are likely to be performed under hypotensive conditions. Controlled hypotension reduces bleeding during surgery. Blood pressure is meticulously monitored during surgeries of all types. When a hypotensive technique is used, a patient's mean arterial pressure (MAP) is reduced, usually to approximately 60 mm Hg. If the MAP drops below 60 mm Hg, evoked potential data can be adversely affected. Because this is a systemic change, cortical as well as sub cortical data will display a decrease. It is very important for the audiologist to keep track of blood pressure throughout a case. If blood pressure values are not known or monitored, a sudden change may result in a false-positive warning to the surgeon.

A patient's body temperature can also affect evoked potential data. Most cases involving SEP monitoring are performed under normal to slightly reduced body temperature. Sudden changes in a patient's temperature are usually unexpected and unwanted by all involved in the surgery. Decreases in a patient's temperature adversely affect evoked potential data. Core temperatures of 34° C or less will result in a decrease or loss of data, peripherally more quickly than cortically. Conversely, our experience with hyperthermia suggests this condition has little to no adverse affect on somatosensory data.

In summary, anesthetic routines are as varied as the personnel involved in their administration. This information only presents general guidelines. Other types of agents, narcotics, or muscle relaxants not mentioned here may be in use in any operative setting. The preceding information regarding dosage and method of administration should still be considered when dealing with a drug in any of the defined categories.

Anesthesia plays an integral role in the successful monitoring of any patient in surgery. The importance of understanding and being familiar with anesthetic protocol cannot be stressed enough. Equally important is the working relationship one must develop with anesthesia personnel. It is the audiologist's responsibility to obtain all necessary information from the anesthesiologist and use this information accordingly. Responsibility also includes informing these same people of our requirements for obtaining consistent, reliable data. (See Table 9–2.)

EQUIPMENT CONSIDERATIONS

Intraoperative monitoring equipment consists of three basic systems: stimulus generation, recording, and data storage. The following discussion addresses the components and functions of these systems.

STIMULUS GENERATION
Constant Current Versus Constant Voltage

Most commercially available systems provide stimulation in either constant voltage or constant current. The audiologist selects the type of stimulus preferred. We prefer the use of constant current for SEP monitoring for a number of reasons.

TABLE 9-2.   ANESTHESIA FOR INTRAOPERATIVE SEP MONITORING.

Drug	Effect on Data SEP	Recommended Dosage/ Administration
Isoflurane Enflurane Halothane Desflurane*	Suppresses cortical responses	0.5% or less endtitle
Nitrous oxide	Suppresses cortical data	50% or less endtitle
Fentanyl Sufentanyl Propofol	Minimal effect if used alone	Drip infusion
Morphine Valium Versed	Suppresses cortical responses	Preop bolus drip infusion intraoperative
Ketamine	Minimal to no effect	Drip infusion
Muscle relaxant	Insufficient dose causes muscle artifact	Repeated bolus to maintain 0 or 1 for four
Arfonad Nitroglycerine Sodium nitroprusside Labatalol	No effect	Dosage to lower pressure to 60 mm Hg

* New inhalation agent, exact recommended dosage not established.

Delivery of constant current allows the audiologist to control the amount of current reaching the patient. Constant current systems adjust voltage to accommodate impedance changes encountered at the stimulation site. If the current level cannot be delivered because of resistance or stimulus artifact, an "impedance limit" or similar message will typically be displayed. The message will be triggered when a stimulating electrode is dislodged or is not in contact with the patient.

Constant current stimulation also allows for a more consistent comparison between evaluations performed at different facilities. When the intensity of a stimulus is known and can be replicated, test results are more comparable.

Constant voltage does not control for impedance at the stimulation site. Therefore, if resistance is low, it is possible to deliver more stimulus than when resistance may be very high. The examiner has no way of knowing exactly what percentage of the stimulus is being delivered to the patient. However, we do recommend purchase of a system with both stimulus options available. Constant voltage is used in other types of evoked potential testing and in other modalities.

Stimulus Rate

Rate of stimulation is another stimulus parameter to be considered. Equipment should allow for adjustment of this parameter. Rate of stimulation refers to the number of stimuli delivered in 1 second. An appropriate rate should allow data collection in a timely manner. If the presentation rate is too fast, morphology of a response may be degraded. If the rate is too slow, data collection becomes too time consuming. We feel use of a rate between 4.1 and 4.7 Hz is optimal. This is used in all types of SEP monitoring (upper and lower limb). Do not make the rate a multiple of 60 Hz, such as 4.0 Hz. This may result in AC current interference from any electrical source in the room.

Stimulus Duration

Duration refers to the effective "on" time of the stimulus. This is another adjustable parameter. We utilize a 0.3 msec duration for most of our intraoperative cases. Patients presenting with "peripheral neuropathy" may produce better SEP data with an increased signal duration, such as 0.5 msec. It is important to remember that longer duration signals increase the intensity of stimulus delivery. The audiologist should adjust stimulus intensity (decreasing) when increasing duration.

A typical situation might be stimulation at 25 mA with 0.3 msec duration. If recordings are of poor quality, an increase in duration to 0.5 msec and decreases in intensity to 20 mA may improve data.

Stimulus Intensity

Intensity level of the stimulus should be of sufficient strength to excite all neurons contained within a nerve. This is sometimes referred to as "the point of maximal stimulation."

An appropriate stimulus intensity level can be determined in several ways. One method involves using an ascending protocol until a motor twitch is found. This intensity, known as the "motor threshold," is doubled and data is collected at that intensity. For example when stimulating the posterior tibial nerve, a motor twitch is seen in the great toe at 13 mA. Taking this value as the "motor threshold," the audiologist would double the intensity of this stimulus and collect data with a stimulating intensity of 26 mA.

Another technique uses an ascending method of stimulus application. Stimulus intensity is increased until a response is observed and then stimulation continues above this level until an increase in stimulus current produces no increase in response amplitude (Figure 9-2).

Our procedure for stimulus intensity selection utilizes elements of both methods. Because motor thresholds are not always obtainable intraoperatively (because of use of muscle relaxants), the method of response detection and doubling is utilized. The stimulation intensity level (in the vast majority of cases), usually falls somewhere between 20 and 30 mA.

Recording System

The recording system includes headboxes, differential amplifiers, band pass filters, and a signal averager. The headbox is the point of connection between the amplifiers and the patient. Equipment specifically designed for use in the operating room is recommended.

Electrical shielding is built into operating room headboxes to protect the patient and the equipment from stray electrical leakage. We strongly urge audiologists to not use accessories designed for diagnostic use in the intraoperative setting.

Differential Amplifiers

Differential amplification reduces the collection of extraneous noise as part of the averaged response. Differential amplifiers receive the signals obtained at the headbox. The activity from the reference and active electrodes at each recording site is summed. The polarity of the reference electrode is reversed. The active electrode polarity remains the same. This "summation" cancels activity that is similar at each site and enhances what is different, namely the SEP signal. A separate amplification system exists for each recording channel.

Filters

The output from the differential amplifier is filtered. Filters are used to selectively enhance the frequency range in which the desired response is to be found. They can be adjusted to eliminate or attenuate frequencies not useful to the response. Filter settings should reflect the characteristics of the responses recorded. In general, slower cortical activity will contain a narrower band of frequencies. Peripheral activity, which is faster in nature, will have a much wider band of frequencies. Filtering must be adjustable for each recording channel.

Cortical, subcortical, and peripheral recording sites are used in intraoperative monitoring. Typically, filters are set for each recording site. An example of bandpass settings for these sites would be:

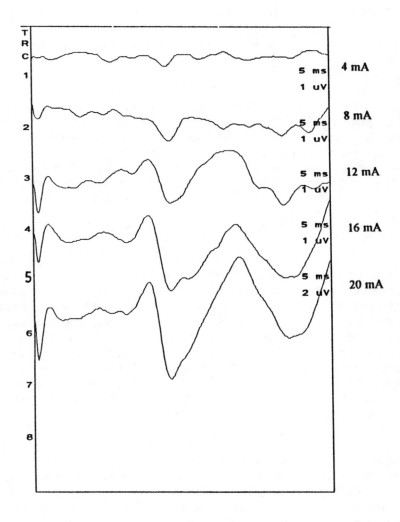

FIGURE 9–2. Response amplitude increases with increasing stimulus intensity.

139

Cortical:	20 Hz to 250 Hz
Subcortical:	20 Hz to 2000 Hz
Peripheral:	20 Hz to 2000 Hz

Each recording channel can then best "capture" the frequencies contained within the response.

Sensitivity

Monitoring equipment allows the user to adjust the sensitivity of the amplifier. Signals that fall outside the selected voltage range are rejected before being averaged. A more sensitive setting results in a greater number of samples that will be rejected. This may increase averaging time. A less sensitive setting will allow an excessive amount of noise to be averaged, possibly obscuring the response. One must consider both aspects when chosing this setting. A sensitivity setting of 10 μv per division for SEP recordings is generally recommended.

Signal Averager

The last component of the monitoring system that enhances the signal-to-noise ratio is the signal averager. Signals that are time-locked to the presentation of the stimulus are converted to a digital signal. The computer captures a set number of samples (we generally use 300 samples) and computes the mean of each data point. This mean is displayed on the monitor as a waveform. The signal-to-noise ratio improves as the noise averages towards zero and the evoked response improves over time. For example, a waveform based on a sample of 1,000 may yield a better morphology than a waveform based on a sample of 100. Unfortunately, a 1,000-sample waveform takes 10 times longer to accumulate and this slow analysis may introduce another set of errors.

Storage System

The storage capabilities of the monitoring system should allow each set of data collected to be stored on the hard computer drive or on a floppy disk. Waveforms, amplitude, and latency measurements should be stored. Most systems utilize a printer to allow immediate production of a hard copy while continuing to monitor and gather more information.

Accessories

There are a few other pieces of accessory equipment that we suggest for intraoperative monitoring.

The first one is a stimulus switching box. Most commercially available equipment provides two or four stimulator inputs. Mixed modality monitoring usually requires multiple stimulation sites (we have used as many as 14 in one case). Ease of access to these sites is greatly improved with a switching box.

Electrodes from all stimulation sites are plugged into the box, which is usually affixed to the operative table at the start of the procedure. The "channel selector" is used to choose the desired stimulation site. In essence, all possible stimulation sites are prepared, plugged in and can be alternated as needed by appropriate manipulation of the channel selector. Some of the manufacturing companies are making this system available. A handheld nerve stimulator is very useful. These are traditionally used by the anesthesiologists to estimate the level of muscle relaxation. They are battery-operated and portable. Nerve stimulators can be used to verify placement of stimulating electrodes when setting up a case and of course allow the audiologist to verify the level of neuromuscular blockade.

Another option that should be considered is partitioning the computer hard drive with a disk operating system. This allows use of the monitoring equipment for report writing, database storage, and so on. Many of the commercially available systems offer this option.

MATERIALS

Electrodes

Any "far field" recording technique requires the use of electrodes for stimulation and recording. There are two types of electrodes commonly used for intraoperative monitoring, surface cup electrodes and subdermal needle electrodes. The advantages and disadvantages of both are discussed.

Surface Electrodes

A standard 3 mm-diameter gold cup electrode is recommended. These should be used for stimulation and recording. Surface electrodes are applied to the patient in the preop holding area. Collodion is a glue-like substance used to attach the electrodes to the patient. Collodion is a highly flammable adhesive that is applied to the electrode site to increase adhesion. Collodion is applied with a cotton- type swab and the cup electrode is placed directly on the collodion. The collodion is allowed to dry (3–5 minutes) before the electrolyte gel is inserted through the hole in the cup electrode to fill the inner electrode space. Impedance of the electrodes is checked and should closely match from one recording site to the other. Periodic rechecking is necessary because the electrolyte can dry out and cause impedance imbalance. When this occurs electrolyte must be reapplied.

Subdermal Electrodes

A 26-gauge, 1.3-cm needle, composed of platinum-iridium, or stainless steel is recommended. Again, it is recommended these be used for stimulation and recording. These needle electrodes are applied after a patient has been anesthetized. Each insertion site is prepped with alcohol. The electrode is inserted through the skin and taped securely in place.

We prefer use of needle electrodes for several reasons. Needle electrodes are quickly and accurately placed within the patient. Surface electrodes require electrolyte, which tends to dry out, increasing impedances and mandating continued maintenance throughout lengthy procedures. When using surface electrodes, impedance must be checked regularly to monitor for electrolyte problems, which must be quickly addressed by reapplication of electrolyte.

Impedances of surface and needle electrodes are inherently different. Surface electrodes, because of their greater area have typically low impedance values when correctly applied. Needle electrodes on the other hand, tend to have fairly high impedance, because the area of the electrode is much smaller. However, interelectrode balance is usually excellent.

Lower impedance is generally preferred for optimal recording of data. Our experience with needle electrodes however, has been very good. Consistent reliable data is recorded with higher impedance values in our experience. Disadvantages to using subdermal electrodes are something to be aware of. Needle electrodes increase the "invasiveness" of the procedure. It is possible for needles to break off within the skin or musculature of the patient. Also, needle electrodes can increase the likelihood of contaminating the patient or the audiologist. For instance, one must consider the possibility of an accidental needle stick after removing needle electrodes from a previously undiagnosed HIV-positive patient. High intensity electrical stimulation may result in a lesion at the insertion site.

If subdermal needle electrodes are used, it is recommended the disposable variety be used. Reusable electrodes must be cleaned and wrapped by someone, increasing the risk of infection. Further, heat methods used to sterilize the cleaned and wrapped electrodes can weaken the electrode, thus increasing the likelihood of breakage. The standard method of heat sterilization is referred to as "autoclave." Ethylene oxide gas sterilization is another option. The primary advantage is that gas process does not damage needles. Importantly, some of the manufacturers of reusable products are reluctant to guarantee product sterility when a gas method is used.

Disposable electrodes solve both of these problems. They come already sterilized and as they are single use, they do not require cleaning, wrapping, or resterilization. The possibility of contamination is greatly reduced with disposable products.

In summary, we prefer needle electrodes. Disposable electrodes provide more safety for both the audiologist and the patient. From our experience, we conclude that disposable needle electrodes are time and cost effective and are the safest way to proceed.

MONITORED PATHWAYS

LOWER EXTREMITY

The primary monitored pathway during spinal surgery is that of the posterior tibial nerve beginning at the level of the medial malleolus. An electrical stimulus of adequate intensity will depolarize the nerve segment, creating an afferent neural volley that can be measured at several locations.

The first recording site is at the level of the popliteal fossa (Figure 9–3). A bipolar recording technique records the action potential as the neural volley passes through this area. Presence of this response confirms that the nerve is being stimulated at an intensity sufficient to evoke recordable potentials further along the neural pathway. Absence of a response at this level suggests that the stimulus intensity or electrode placement is inadequate or that the patient has peripheral neurologic disorder, such as peripheral neuropathy or neural injury that precludes normal conduction of the nerve segment.

The neural volley ascends the posterior tibial nerve to a larger nerve bundle, the sciatic nerve, just proximal to the knee. The sciatic nerve bundle then enters the pelvis where it divides into smaller nerve bundles called nerve roots. Each nerve root enters or exits the spinal canal at a separate neural foramen, located between each vertebral body. The neural volley originating from innervation of the posterior tibial nerve enters the spinal canal through the foramen at spinal levels L4 through S1.

The neural volley ascends ipsilaterally, primarily through the posterior columns of the spinal cord. The synapse of fibers at the cervicomedullary junction can be recorded at 28 msec after stimulation at the level of the medial malleolus (Figure 9–4).

The volley continues its ascent and crosses to the contralateral side, through the thalamus and to the sensory cortical area. The polyphasic cortical response is generated from the midline sensory cortical area approximately 40 msec following stimulation at the medial malleolus.

The peroneal nerve can be stimulated at the lateral side of the knee at the fibular head. From here, the nerve extends to the posterior thigh, where it joins the sciatic. The afferent volley created in the peroneal nerve enters the spinal canal at the L4 through S2 spinal levels. The femoral nerve is stimulated in the lateral aspect of the groin at the inguinal ligament. The proper stimulus site

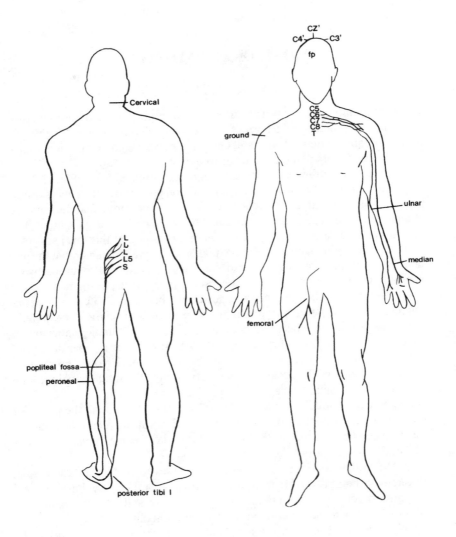

FIGURE 9–3. Stimulating and recording sites.

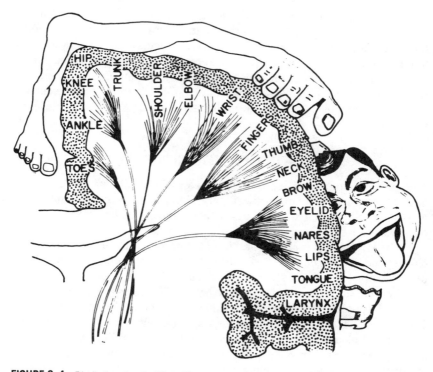

FIGURE 9–4. Distribution of cortical fibers. The lower extremity fibers are located at the midline, and upper extremity fibers are lateral.

is easily determined by palpating the femoral artery, as the nerve follows this course. The femoral nerve enters the spinal canal at the L2, L3, and L4 spinal levels. From this point, the afferent volley in both the peroneal and femoral nerves parallels that of the posterior tibial. See Figure 9–3 for illustration of stimulus and recording sites.

UPPER EXTREMITY

The median and ulnar nerves of the upper extremities are used to monitor function of the brachial plexus and cervical spine during spine surgery. The median nerve is stimulated at the wrist. The ulnar nerve can be stimulated at the wrist or the cubital tunnel (see Figure 9–3). The afferent volley can be recorded in a series of potentials. The first occurs peripherally in the brachial plexus approximately 9 msec following stimulation at the wrist. Potentials can be recorded from the cervical spine at approximately 11 and 13 msec, generated by fibers synapsing at the root entry zone and at the cervicomedullary junction. Following this, crossover of fibers occurs and the volley ascends to the sensory cortical areas. The cortical response occurs approximately 20 msec after stimulation at the sensory cortical area contralateral to the extremity stimulated (Figure 9-4). Stimulation of the ulnar nerve at the cubital tunnel will generate potentials shorter in latency than those from the level of the wrist.

STIMULATION SITES

The most important and appropriate sites for stimulation are related to the neurologic structures involved in a surgery. Upper and lower limb stimulation is used for all monitored spinal cases. Our protocol uses primary and secondary stimulation sites.

If a surgical site is at vertebral level C7 or above, the upper limbs, specifically median and ulnar nerves, will be the primary stimulation sites and the posterior tibial nerve will serve as the secondary site.

When a surgery involves the spine below C7, nerves in the lower limbs, such as the posterior tibial and femoral nerve will serve as primary sites. (See Table 9-3.) The reasons for utilizing these specific nerves are anatomical. The median and ulnar nerves are most sensitive to events in the cervical spine, although the posterior tibial nerve is always used to provide additional information concerning the spinal cord.

Cases involving the more distal segments of the spinal cord and spinal column require primary stimulation sites in the lower limbs. The posterior tibial nerve is an excellent choice. The femoral nerve is stimulated in cases involving lumbosacral segments of the spine. It can be sensitive to position related deficits and muscle injury related to retractor pressure.

Secondary stimulation sites have a variety of uses. They provide the examiner with an indication of systemic function. For example, a case involving the thoracic spine would have the posterior tibial nerves as the primary stimulation sites. A secondary site, such as the median nerve, can provide useful information about anesthetic variables in the event data were degraded or lost from the posterior tibial sites. Another reason to use the secondary stimulation site is to provide additional information concerning the integrity of the spinal cord. As stated previously, upper and lower limbs are monitored during all surgeries. In addition to sensitivity of cervical spine function, upper limb stimulation and monitoring allows assessment of brachial plexus function. Improper positioning of a patient on the operating table can result in compression to nerves in the brachial plexus. Additional factors such as intraoperative halo traction ("halo" type ring affixed to patient's skull with various

TABLE 9–3. STIMULATION SITES.

Surgical Spinal Level	Primary Stimulation Sites	Secondary Stimulation Sites
Cervical spine	Median nerve Ulnar nerve	Posterior tibial nerve
Thoracic spine	Posterior tibial nerve	Median/ulnar nerves Peroneal nerve
Lumbar spine	Posterior tibial nerve Femoral nerve	Median/ulnar nerve Peroneal nerve
Sacral spine	Posterior tibial nerve Femoral nerve	Median/ulnar nerve Peroneal nerve

amounts of weight attached to increase extension or flexion of thoracic and cervical spine) and prolonged surgery can also increase the risk of iatrogenic injury. Median and ulnar nerve data are sensitive to compression of the plexus or peripheral nerves in the upper limbs (OBrien, Lenke, Padberg, Bridwell, & Stokes, 1993).

RECORDING SITES

Our monitoring protocol typically involves four recording channels proximal to the site of surgery. Additionally, peripheral recording sites are utilized. These include:

Cortical = C3′ TO FpZ = Channel 1
            CZ TO FpZ = Channel 2
            C4′ TO FpZ = Channel 3
Subcortical = CRV TO FpZ = Channel 4
Peripheral = Popliteal fossa, bilaterally, median/ulnar nerve in the axilla bilaterally

Cortical sites allow the examiner to view the SEP responses in entirety, from point of stimulation to the somatosensory cortex. A cervical (or non-cortical) site provides data sensitive to surgical events, but less influenced by general anesthesia (Figure 9–5). Peripheral sites are utilized to give information concerning encoding of the response and help to confirm correct placement of stimulating electrodes.

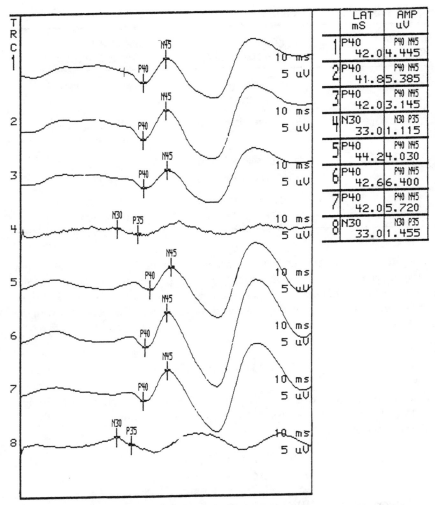

	LAT mS	AMP uV
1	P40 42.0	P40 N45 4.445
2	P40 41.8	P40 N45 5.385
3	P40 42.0	P40 N45 3.145
4	N30 33.0	N30 P35 1.115
5	P40 44.2	P40 N45 4.030
6	P40 42.6	P40 N45 6.400
7	P40 42.0	P40 N45 5.720
8	N30 33.0	N30 P35 1.455

FIGURE 9–5.   Normal posterior tibial nerve response using the three cortical, one cervical recording methodology.

We urge the use of multiple recording sites for intra operative monitoring for a variety of reasons. Multiple cortical sites provide information across the somatosensory cortex. CZ' is the standard recording site used to demonstrate the SEP from the lower limbs. However, inclusion of C3' and C4' provides additional cortical information, increasing the reliability of data. Cortical data is subject to interference from anesthesia and individual patient-related variables. The redundancy of more than one recording site in this area provides additional confirmation of stimulus reception. Also, in some patients C3' and C4' may prove to be larger in amplitude, more consistent and easier to detect responses than the responses recorded from CZ' in some patients (Cruse, Klem, Lesser, & Lueders, 1982).

Subcortical recordings offer unique advantages when used in tandem with cortical responses. As mentioned earlier, subcortical responses are more resistant to anesthetic effects. As such, they are useful in difficult cases, as subcortical data allow confirmation of stimulus and continuity of the signal to a site above the surgical field. In a case where the cortical responses disappear, it is useful to observe the subcortical response as it may offer a clue as to the cortical attenuation being an anesthetic induced false-positive or perhaps an event more likely to be deleterious.

It is recommended that cortical, subcortical, and peripheral recording sites be used in all spinal cases with intraoperative monitoring. The combination of these sites provides the most complete analysis of the structures at-risk (Chiappa, & Ropper 1982). (See Figure 9-3.)

Appropriate use of a ground electrode is also part of the recording system. We always use a ground plate, either disposable or reusable, for all SEP monitoring. Needle electrodes should not be used as a ground, as greater surface area is required to minimize the risk of patient injury at the ground site. Disposable ground plates are prepasted with electrolyte; reusable types require application of some form of conductive gel or cream. Either is appropriate for monitoring. The ground electrodes should always be placed at a point between the stimulating and recording leads. The patient's shoulder is appropriate for most cases.

PREOPERATIVE CONCERNS

As is true in all aspects of audiology, a case history and knowledge of the surgical procedure is highly recommended before entering the operating room. Patient history, diagnosis and surgical procedure are the guidelines that determine appropriate evoked potential methods.

An excellent working relationship must be established with all members of the surgical team. The audiologist and the surgeon must be perfectly "in sync" for expedient interpretation and action based upon data obtained during surgery. The audiologist must also work and communicate effectively with the anesthesiologist in to maintain correct analysis assumptions during surgery.

Certainly, the audiologist needs to understand the case history, presenting symptoms, and surgical plan to determine the most appropriate intraoperative stimulation and recording protocol.

PREOPERATIVE ASSESSMENT

Patients with a history of peripheral neuropathy, circulatory disorders, spinal cord injury, or neuromuscular disease should be "red flagged" as possible candidates for preoperative SEP or dermatomal assessment. A diagnostic evaluation allows the audiologist to determine general characteristics and morphology of a patient's responses before surgery.

If, for example, a patient with diabetic peripheral neuropathy displays poor posterior tibial nerve evoked potentials following stimulation at the ankle, recordings may be significantly improved with stimulation of the nerve at the popliteal fossa. Diagnostic assessment before surgery allows for appropriate preparation. Even more important is the use of preoperative assessment to identify a patient who will not yield any consistent data. Some neuromuscular disorders preclude reliable SEP and neurogenic motor evoked potentials (NMEP) recordings.

Spinal cord injuries and lesions may severely inhibit or alter the evoked potential data. When a preoperative diagnostic study yields poor results, it may be assumed that data collected intraoperatively will likely be poor or worse. Somatosensory testing on an awake, cooperative patient will generally result in optimal data. The effects of anesthesia and the surgical procedure will typically degrade whatever response is obtained in an awake patient.

OPERATING ROOM SETUP

What follows is a step-by-step guide for preparing equipment and setting up the patient in the operating room.

BEFORE THE PATIENT ARRIVES

1. Always be in the operating room 15–30 minutes before the patient arrives.
2. Position the equipment in the operating room. Avoid power sources with multiple outlets whenever possible.
3. Start a patient data file and complete the patient information.
4. Place stimulating and recording equipment in appropriate places (either on or underneath operative table).
5. Connect equipment to the main unit and tape all cables securely to the floor.
6. Prepare (unwrap and uncoil) the number of electrodes you will need for the case. These may be placed in a sterile towel until ready for use.
7. Prepare alcohol swabs, one roll of tape, and a handheld nerve stimulator. These items should be kept handy.

8. If you have not done so previously, check with the surgeon regarding the patient's status and what is being planned for the case.

AFTER THE PATIENT ARRIVES

Placing Stimulating Electrodes

1. Once the patient has been anesthetized but before the patient is paralyzed, place lower limb stimulating electrodes.
2. Check placement with handheld stimulator for an appropriate muscle twitch; reposition electrodes if necessary.
3. When twitches are obtained, inform the anesthesiologist so he or she may proceed with relaxant.
4. Secure electrodes with tape. Coil the leads and place around the patient's toes (provides strain relief).
5. Any other lower limb electrodes should be placed starting with the most distal location and working proximally.
6. Electrodes for the upper limbs should be placed. Median nerve at the wrist, ulnar nerve at the elbow. The elbow may be the most accessible site at this time as the wrist area is reserved for I.V. and arterial lines.
7. Position electrodes and tape securely.
8. Coil the leads and tape to the forearm.
9. A ground electrode should be placed on the deltoid of the arm that will be closest to the recording unit when the patient is positioned for surgery. Coil this lead and tape it to the shoulder.

Placing Recording Electrodes

1. Once the patient has been intubated, cortical leads can be placed. Measure the midpoint between inion and nasion and place CZ electrode 2½ cm posterior to this point (International 10–20 system of electrode placement) (Harner & Sannit, 1974; Jasper, 1958).
2. C1′ and C2′ electrodes are positioned 2-cm lateral on either side of CZ′ for lower limb primary recording.
3. When upper limbs are the primary recording sites, C3′ and C4′ should be utilized.
4. FpZ should be placed and taped. All four leads can be coiled and tucked under the patient's surgical cap. If a cap is not worn, tape the leads to the patient's shoulder.

As the patient is positioned or turned onto the operating table, stand at his or her feet. Be attentive to positioning/turning the patient to ensure the electrodes stay in place. When the patient is in position on the table, plug in the stimulating electrodes. (We begin with the left side, placing these electrodes in odd-numbered inputs, the right side in even-numbered inputs.)

Peripheral recording sites are placed in each popliteal fossa. These should be plugged into a recording unit.

Extender cables may be needed for some stimulating electrodes to reach the stimulus box. Tape excess cable to the side or bottom of the table. This will help prevent the electrodes from being dislodged during the surgical procedure. Check electrode placement in both arms, as turning the patient will sometimes cause the electrodes to become dislodged.

Cortical leads should be plugged into the recording unit. The cervical lead can also be placed. (We find placement immediately distal to the occiput the most consistently located site for a cervical lead.) Plug the ground electrode into the recording unit. Make sure the unit is affixed securely to the operative table and away from anesthetic paraphenalia, especially liquid dripping from an I.V. line.

Verify all stimulation sites before incision. (Start with the primary stimulation sites.) Getting complete averages for all sites may not be possible as the patient is being prepped and draped for surgery. However it is important to verify electrode placement, stimulation, and the presence of a response at all sites. These data should be stored and recorded on your log sheet (See Figure 9-6).

If you find problems when checking sites, correct them right away. Once a patient is prepped and draped for surgery, it becomes more difficult to access all electrode sites.

Inform the surgeon as soon as all preincision data is obtained. (Be very clear about this being preincision and not baseline data.) Abnormalities should be reported with the understanding that further information will be given when baselines are obtained.

Consult with the anesthesia personnel. (Find out what is being used and why.) Record this information on the log sheet. Emphasize to the anesthesiologist the importance of informing you of anesthetic changes made during the procedure.

Baseline data should be obtained after incision is complete, but prior to surgical maneuvers. Record the levels of all anesthetic agents in use, the patient's blood pressure, CO_2, and core temperature at this time. Each of these variables are components of the baseline. (See Figure 9-6.)

SURGICAL MONITORING

RESPONSE CHARACTERISTICS

The somatosensory evoked potential recorded with mixed nerve stimulation such as the posterior tibial nerve will display certain morphological charac-

INTRAOPERATIVE RECORD

NAME:_____DATE:_____SEX:_____D.O.B.:_____INSTR:_____

SURGEON:_____HOSPITAL:_____SPINAL INSTR:_____

PROCEDURE:_____

ANESTHESIA:_____

COMMENTS:_____

SITE:_____					SITE:_____			
LEFT		RIGHT			LEFT		RIGHT	
LAT	AMP	LAT	AMP		LAT	AMP	LAT	AMP
C3 ____	____	____	____		__ ____	____	____	____
CZ ____	____	____	____		__ ____	____	____	____
C4 ____	____	____	____		__ ____	____	____	____
CV ____	____	____	____		__ ____	____	____	____
__ ____	____	____	____		__ ____	____	____	____

SITE:_____					SITE:_____			
LEFT		RIGHT			LEFT		RIGHT	
LAT	AMP	LAT	AMP		LAT	AMP	LAT	AMP
__ ____	____	____	____		__ ____	____	____	____
__ ____	____	____	____		__ ____	____	____	____

FILE   EVENT   TIME

_____
_____
_____
_____
_____
_____
_____
_____
_____
_____
_____
_____
_____
_____
_____
_____
_____

FIGURE 9–6. Intraoperative record.

teristics. The primary response is often referred to as the "P40," the first positive wave occurring at or around 40 msec, recorded from the somatosensory cortex. This nomenclature extends to upper limb responses, the "N20," the first negative wave occurring at or around 20 msec. These terms are only references, the literature also uses "N1, P1, P45, N22," and so on. What is important to understand is that these terms, whatever they may be, are used to signify the presence of a response to stimulation.

The initial marking indicator serves to identify the latency of the response. This indicates the time at which, following stimulation, a response occurs. The latency of a response is a function of the distance between these two points (stimulation and recording points).

A second latency indicator follows and is represented as opposite in polarity from the first. For instance, the P40 is followed by the N50. The second latency marker provides the differential measure from which peak to peak amplitude is determined. Amplitude is measured in millivolts (mV) or microvolts (μv). In a healthy, nonimpaired individual, response amplitude increases (to a maximal response) as stimulus intensity increases.

An example of a normal posterior tibial nerve response for left and right lower limbs is shown in Figure 9–5. Four recordings are pictured for each limb. The responses labeled C3′, CZ′, and C4′ are cortical, the response labeled CRV is the cervical or subcortical. The three cortical responses display a fairly smooth, longer response. This is typical for this type of recording. Cortical activity tends to be "slower" than more peripheral activity. The cervical response displays a sharper, more succinct pattern. This example displays response negativity as an upward deflection and positivity as downward. SEP activity in the cortex manifests its dipole orientation as negative. Therefore, all of our SEP responses are recorded to reflect this orientation.

All evoked potential data must meet certain criteria to be classified as a response (Jones, Howard, & Shawkat, 1988; Owen, Bridwell, & Shimon, 1988). General guidelines include:

1. Appropriate response morphology.
2. Test/retest reliability of latency and amplitude. Latency agreement should not differ by more than 10%, amplitude should be within 30% from one trial to the next.
3. Barring the presence of known pathology, interlimb differences should not exceed 50% in amplitude.
4. Presence of an evoked potential should be verified by use of a "silent control." A response is averaged without stimulus and the resultant tracing is compared to the response obtained with stimulus. This can be accomplished by simply turning stimulus intensity to zero milliamps. The response

obtained with stimulus should exceed the silent control by at least 50% to be considered valid (Owen, 1991).

Latency and amplitude are the response characteristics most important in SEP recordings. Morphology of a response is another term often used in relation to the SEP. This is somewhat more subjective and can be used more as a descriptive term than an objective measure. It refers to the shape of a given response. Certain morphological characteristics are believed to be an indicator of underlying pathology, such as diabetic neuropathy or multiple sclerosis. "Normal" morphology refers to the generally accepted appearance of SEP responses from various stimulation and recording sites.

The literature is replete with recommendations for criteria of significant change in intraoperative monitoring (Jones, Howard, & Shawkat, 1988; Keith, Stambough, & Awender, 1990; Owen, 1991). Many of the recommended procedures have merit. The set of standards identified here is based on experience in hundreds of intraoperative cases as well as review of the literature. We use a 10% or greater increase in latency and or a 60% or greater decrease in amplitude as criteria for significant change. These values must deviate from baselines established during surgery.

Interpretation of data requires using the above stated criteria. We generally regard amplitude as the primary indicator of change (Owen, 1991). Latency is always utilized, but research suggests it to be less sensitive to surgical events.

DATA INTERPRETATION

CRITERIA

This section deals with one of the most important aspects of intraoperative monitoring. There is no set of "normative data for o.r. monitoring" on any given patient. In effect, each patient serves as his or her own control. The responses obtained as baselines for each individual should be "normal" for the duration of that surgery. Obviously, general guidelines, such as those listed previously are useful in determining if things are approximately as they should be or if a gross abnormality is present.

What must be understood is that perisurgical variables such as wound temperature, body temperature, MAP, and anesthesia affects each patient differently. A common mistake made by audiologists new to this field is to infer from what is seen and learned from one case over to the next.

Obviously, previous experience will be of tremendous help in identifying problems and dealing with them appropriately. One must remember, however, to regard each case as a situation unto itself. Do not expect the same pattern of events to occur just because a surgical procedure is similar. Try not to approach your cases with preconceived notions or expectations.

BASELINES

Baselines are obtained at the completion of the surgical incision, before any maneuvers are performed (correction of deformity, tumor removal, etc.) that would place the neural structure(s) at risk for injury. "Baselines" obtained before this time are not true measures of the patient's status, but are instead a confirmation of stimulation and recording integrity. Multiple trials can be obtained and an average of values taken as baseline data. This provides the audiologist with more representative measures to compare later data to. Caution is advised in spending too much time in the averaging of many trials. The surgical procedure is ongoing and baselines must be established for all stimulation sites prior to any surgical event.

All baseline information should be recorded on the intraoperative record (see Figure 9–6). This serves as the reference for all future data collected. All log entries should include time of acquisition. It is also helpful to chart progress of the surgical procedure with each entry. Anesthetic changes should be indicated on the log sheet along with time of occurrence.

WHEN TO MONITOR

Each surgical procedure will have critical times for monitoring. It is important that the audiologist be aware of these and prepare accordingly. Minimally, data should be obtained at the following points during a case:

1. Prior to incision/postintubation.
2. Postincision baselines.
3. Immediately prior to any procedure putting structures at-risk.
4. Continuously during critical times.
5. Continuously, for at least 30 minutes following the last maneuver placing any structure at risk.
6. Just prior to final closure of wound.
7. At regular intervals during other noncrucial times.

The pathways most sensitive to surgical variables are monitored exclusively during critical points of a surgery. Secondary stimulation sites are monitored less often; for example, data for brachial plexus function may be obtained every 30 minutes, while primary sites are continuously monitored.

Data from all recording sites sensitive to surgical maneuver must demonstrate change. For example, if amplitude is reduced by 60% or more from a posterior tibial nerve response, this reduction must be apparent at all recording sites, cortical and subcortical. Also, if latency increases by 10% or more, the increase must be seen for all sites. Guidelines for verifying a change and notification of the surgeon are outlined below. These guidelines and possible modifications should be discussed with the surgeon before the surgery begins. It is critical that the surgeon is fully informed and in agreement with what the reporting protocol will be.

Discuss the monitoring procedure and protocol with your surgeon before a case. Make sure you are both very clear on what the policy is going to be if data change significantly. Procedural guidelines are:

1. A test run indicates a reportable change.
2. Retest. If retest demonstrates the same problem, check a peripheral recording site to verify encoding of the response. For example, lost tibial data requires a check of the response recording at the popliteal fossa.
3. Verify impedance from all recording sites.
4. Check data from another stimulation site, one that would not be sensitive to surgical variables to verify systemic function.
5. Consult anesthesia personnel. Determine if any changes have occurred in use of agent, narcotic, and so on. Verify patient's temperature and mean arterial pressure.
6. Inform surgeon of change.

Informing the surgeon of a change in the SEP indicates that you, as the audiologist, have eliminated the possibility of any technical component or anesthetic variable as being responsible for the change in data. It is *extremely important* to check equipment and anesthetics in a **time efficient manner**. If the data demonstrate true positive changes, an adjustment of surgical technique or removal of instrumentation may reverse the problem, if accomplished in time.

To inform the surgeon, make sure you have the physician's full attention. Be concise and to the point about which stimulation and recording sites are demonstrating a problem and when this was first noted. It will be very helpful to have a good grasp of what was happening surgically when the change was first noted. Make sure the surgeon verbally responds to the information. A log entry is necessary that includes time of events, the nature of the event, and the time and nature of the surgeon's notification and response.

Once a warning has been given the following steps may occur:

1. The surgeon does nothing and continues working.
2. The surgeon will stop all activity, wait for 5 minutes and ask you to check data again.

3. All activity stops, any instrumentation is removed, and a wake-up test is ordered.
4. The surgeon orders a wake-up test, but continues with the surgical procedure.

After a surgeon has responded to your warning, monitoring must continue. A wake-up test will usually take up to 20 minutes to perform. This involves reversal of muscle relaxant and sedation, bringing a patient to a level of conciousness allowing the individual to respond to verbal commands. The patient is asked to move upper and lower extremities. Personnel in the operating room will observe the subsequent activity. It is important to continue to monitor, because the rise in blood pressure during a wake-up will sometimes improve data. The surgeon should be kept informed of the status of the responses throughout this time. All information pertaining to the wake-up test should be recorded on the log sheet.

Always remember the limits of your responsibility. Provide the surgeon with all information regarding the structures monitored. Inform the physician about any significant change in a timely fashion and do everything within your scope to provide the most reliable, accurate assessment of the patient's neurologic status during the particular surgery.

TROUBLESHOOTING

The following chart (Table 9–4) lists possible problems encountered during intraoperative monitoring and methods for pinpointing and alleviating them.

DERMATOMAL SOMATOSENSORY EVOKED POTENTIALS

Dermatomal somatosensory evoked potentials (DSEP) differ from mixed nerve potentials in that the cutaneous fibers rather than a large nerve branch are stimulated to evoke a response. A dermatome is an area of skin that is supplied by fibers of a single spinal nerve root (Stedman's, 1990).

The dermatomal fields and their related spinal levels are illustrated in Figure 9-7. Discrete stimulation of a single dermatomal field can provide information regarding the conduction ability of the individual spinal nerve from which it receives innervation. In contrast, mixed nerves receive innervation from several spinal levels, hence the evoked potentials they generate may not be sensitive to an abnormality at a single spinal level. To illustrate, Figure 9-8 demonstrates a herniated intervertebral disc compressing the left L5 spinal root as it passes through the neural foramen. Despite the compression,

TABLE 9–4. TROUBLESHOOTING GUIDE.

Problem	Possible Solutions
1. No response	Check stimulation electrodes Check amplifiers Check encoding with peripheral site
2. Poor cortical data	Check with anesthesia Verify lead placement
3. Poor cervical data	Check level of relaxant Verify lead placement
4. Input rejection	Verify recording sites Check ground Check level of relaxant Decrease amplifier sensitivity
5. Poor response	Verify stimulating leads Increase intensity Increase duration of stimulus Stimulate more proximally
6. "Impedance limit" message	Check stimulating electrodes Check all points of connection between patient and equipment
7. Excessive noise in any traces	Separate recording leads from any other monitoring equipment Change rate of stimulation Check other electrical equipment in operating room

the peroneal and posterior tibial nerve EPs are normal (Figure 9–9). This "false negative" outcome occurs because both mixed nerves have healthy fibers extending from spinal levels other than L5 that contribute to the evoked response. However, the specific fibers yielding the left L5 DSEP travel through the affected foramen, resulting in an abnormal response (Figure 9–9).

METHOD

Use of tab electrodes is recommended for stimulation rather than cup or subdermal types. A 22 × 32 mm tab (Nicolet Biomedical) has the ability to

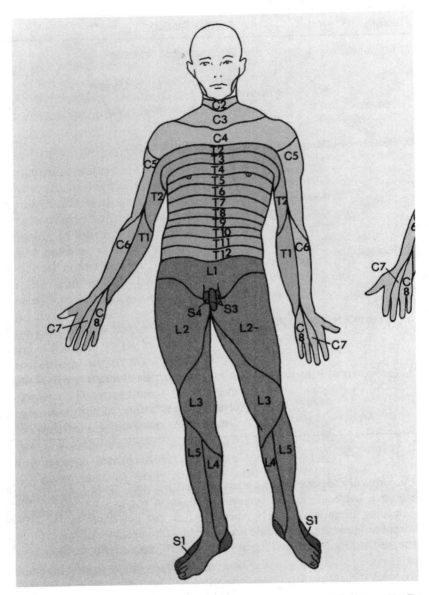

FIGURE 9–7. Dermatomal segments. (From Weinreb, Eva Lurie, *Anatomy and Physiology,* 1984, The Addison Wesley Publishing Company. Reprinted with permission.

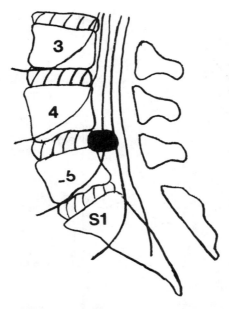

FIGURE 9–8. Compression of the L5 nerve root by a herniated intervertebral disc.

stimulate a large surface area, recruiting a great number of cutaneous fibers. Care should be taken to apply stimulating electrodes in an area of the dermatomal field least likely to result in current spread and the resultant recruitment of fibers from adjacent dermatomes. Figures 9–10 and 9–11 indicate optimal stimulus sites. Stimulus intensity should be applied using an ascending method, noting the level required for sensory threshold and the level that is determined by the patient as being strong but not painful. This level is typically between 10 and 25 mA and should be at least twice that of the sensory threshold. Sensory threshold and test level for each site should be recorded.

A polyphasic potential is measured from the somatosensory cortical areas. C3' and C4' are the active recording locations used for upper extremity responses, CZ' for the lower extremity responses. FPZ is used as the referent location, the shoulder as the ground. Three hundred samples should be obtained, using a bandpass of 10 to 250 Hz, with amplifier sensitivity of 10 microvolts per division. Intraoperatively, higher intensity levels are required than those used in the diagnostic setting. Typically 25 to 30 mA is adequate using a pulse width of 0.3 msec. Observe the waveform for signs of fatigue

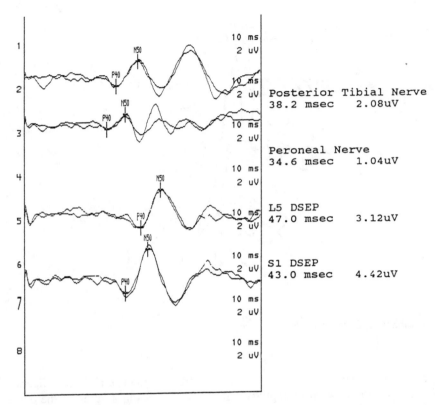

FIGURE 9-9. Normal posterior tibial and peroneal SEPs; however, the L5 DSEP latency is delayed relative to S1.

such as deterioration of the response amplitude and reduce intensity, if necessary. DSEP response latencies are similar to mixed nerve response latencies of the same extremity. Response latency is a function of the distance of the dermatomal field from the recording site. Response amplitude is dependent on stimulus intensity.

Every dermatomal field cannot be reliably utilized for spinal nerve root evaluation because the size and configuration may prohibit reliable placement of stimulating electrodes. In addition, comparison of published dermatomal fields reveals overlap and inconsistency among authors (Figure 9-12). Those dermatomal fields that are most consistently identified and have suitable size and configuration are C5 through C8 and L2 through S1. Each of the stimulus sites in Figures 9-10 and 9-11 allows adequate placement of the tab electrodes. Ring electrodes are effective when stimulating the derma-

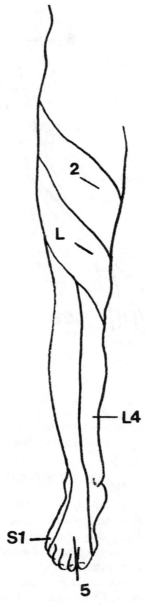

FIGURE 9–10. LS–S1 DSEP stimulus sites.

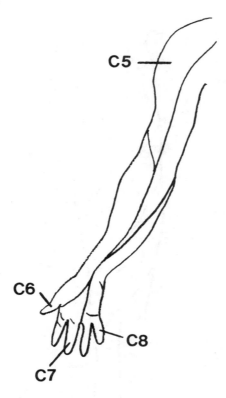

FIGURE 9–11. C5–C8 DSEP stimulus sites.

tomes of the digits. Be certain that ring electrodes are not so tight as to cause compression injury yet are tight enough not to slide off the finger.

INTERPRETIVE CRITERIA

DSEPs tend to demonstrate morphology that is not as robust and reliable as mixed nerve responses. This is exacerbated further by anesthetic affects. DSEPs collected intraoperatively may demonstrate significant moment-to-moment variability that is unrelated to surgical manipulation. Because of this, the standard criteria for significant change intraoperatively is total absence of a response that was present earlier in the procedure.

Reliable data can be routinely obtained from the awake, cooperative patient. Therefore, interpretation of a diagnostic DSEP evaluation differs significantly from intraoperative interpretation. It requires measurement of the

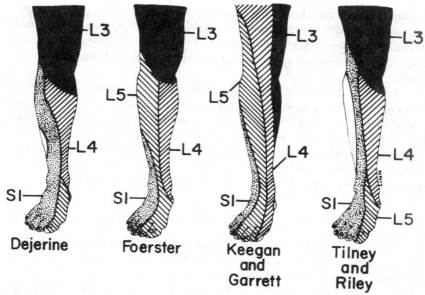

FIGURE 9–12. Variability among published dermatomal charts.

P1 latency and the P1 to N1 peak-to-peak amplitude of each dermatomal response. Three trials for each dermatome should be compared to assure repeatability of latency and amplitude. After responses from all dermatomal fields are collected, they are compared to the other DSEPs from the same patient. Using this interpretive method, variables such as height and age apparent in normative data are not at issue. The criteria for abnormality are:

1. Interside latency difference at the same neurologic level greater than 3 msec (the later response is abnormal).
2. Interside amplitude difference at the same neurologic level greater than 50% (the smaller response is abnormal). It is important to verify that the same or similar intensity levels have been used.
3. Ipsilateral latencies should be sequential, moving proximal to distal, such as: L2 latency should occur before L3, L3 prior to L4, and so on.

APPLICATION

Intervertebral disc degeneration and the resultant spinal instability or trauma are typical conditions in which the conduction of spinal nerves is affected.

Collapse of disc space height from disc degeneration or spinal deformity and the subsequent spread of disc material results in narrowing of the spinal canal or neural foramen through which the nerve roots pass. Compression of nerve fibers causes peripheral symptoms of numbness, pain, and weakness in the extremities they serve.

Intraoperatively, DSEPs provide information of the conduction integrity of the spinal nerve roots. Surgically, the intent is to effectively decompress the neural structures and in some cases, reestablish disc space height through the use of bone graft with or without instrumentation. Typical cases where DSEPs are useful are cervical or lumbar discectomies and laminectomies. DSEPs can provide useful information of the conduction integrity of each nerve root preoperatively, potentially aiding in surgical planning.

LIMITATIONS

As in any neurophysiologic test, DSEPs have limitations. First, the afferent neural volley cannot be recorded reliably peripherally. Therefore, they are measured from the scalp only. As it is a one-channel recording, the DSEP reflects the conduction ability of the entire pathway and cannot definitively pinpoint the exact location of a conduction blockage. For example, DSEPs cannot differentiate compression of an L4 spinal nerve root in the spinal canal versus the neural foramen. Diagnostic DSEPs should be used in conjunction with the information derived from anatomic studies such as MRI or CT scans.

Second, the type of anesthesia greatly affects the reliability of intraoperative DSEPs. A typical balanced narcotic technique may allow recording of mixed nerve evoked potentials, yet can diminish or eliminate DSEPs. A ketamine-based technique has been suggested as optimal for recording DSEPs (Owen et al., 1991). Use of propofol may also provide a good recording environment; however, its specific use with DSEP recording has not been investigated. Third, adequate surgical decompression of a nerve root will not routinely result in improvement of DSEP latency or amplitude (Owen et al., 1991). Frequently, DSEPs will deteriorate intraoperatively following decompression because of irritation of the nerve root and the edema caused by surgical manipulation.

Because of these shortfalls, it is recommended that DSEPs be utilized as a secondary SEP modality. The more robust mixed nerve responses should serve as the primary pathway monitored. However, despite the intraoperative limitations, there is clear utility to DSEPs, particularily in the diagnosis.

MOTOR EVOKED POTENTIALS

A major risk of surgeries of the spine is damage to neural tissue resulting in paralysis. Intraoperative monitoring of SEPs has been the "gold standard" in protecting the spinal cord. However, SEPs evaluate only the sensory tracts of the spinal cord. There are reports of unchanged intraoperative SEPs in patients demonstrating postoperative motor deficits (Lesser et al., 1986; Mustain & Kendig, 1991; Ben-David, Haller, & Taylor, 1987). Because of these false negative reports, research has been focused on the development of methods to monitor the motor pathways of the spinal cord.

The motor cortex lies posterior to the sensory cortical area. Information from the motor cortex to the peripheries is transmitted along the corticospinal tract, posterolaterally through the spinal cord to the anterior horn cells. The descending messages are transmitted to the muscles in the extremities by way of the peripheral nerves.

Much work has been completed researching electrical or magnetic stimulation applied to the motor cortex through the skull. However, despite somewhat promising results, these methods have not become mainstream in the clinical setting. Typically, a large current is required for adequate motor cortex stimulation, resulting in stimulation of other area of the brain and jerking of the extremities. Changes in EEG activity have been reported (Hufnagel et al., 1989) following cortical stimulation and it is not recommended for patients with a history of seizures.

Direct stimulation of the spinal cord avoids the problems inherent to cortical stimulation and has been successfully utilized to measure spine-to-spine potentials or spine-to periphery potentials (Tamaki, 1984). Epidural electrodes are used for stimulation proximal to the surgical site; a response is recorded from the spinal cord in the distal portion of the wound. Or, an evoked myogenic response can be recorded from the muscle groups in the lower extremities. The drawback to epidural placement is inadvertent movement of the stimulating or recording electrodes in the wound, which would result in changes of the stimulus level or the amplitude of the responses. In some cases, the surgical exposure may not be extensive enough to accomodate epidural placement. In addition, recording of electromyogenic activity is often contrary to the needs of the surgeon, who requires a relaxed patient.

NEUROGENIC MOTOR EVOKED POTENTIALS

Owen, Laschinger, Bridwell, Shimon, & Nielsen (1988) describe a method of recording a motor evoked potential that eliminates the need for placement of electrodes on the dura and allows the anesthesiologist to use a neuromuscular blockade for relaxation. Stimulation is applied to the spinal cord and the efferent neural volley is recorded from the nerves in the extremities. The response is recorded prior to the neuromuscular junction; therefore, it is neurogenic in nature. This technique involves placement of 1.3 cm, 23 gauge stimulating electrodes into adjacent spinous processes in the proximal wound. The surgeon removes the tip of the process to allow placement of the electrodes into cancellous bone. An alternative is placement at the base of the process. Either way, the tip of the electrode should be approximately 1 cm from the spinal cord. In both placements, as the electrodes are sunk deep into bone, chances of dislodging them are slim.

Stimulation is applied using an ascending method. typically the response is recordable following stimulus levels of 50 to 150 V. Adequate responses can be obtained from the sciatic notch or from the popliteal fossa using the same electrodes utilized for SEP recording (Figure 9–13).

An alternative stimulus site when recording NMEPs that is less invasive than the spinous process placement is percutaneous placement of stimulating electrodes proximal to the sterile field. In this method, 6 cm electrodes coated in Teflon except for the tip are inserted through the skin at the posterior cervical spine. To ensure safety, electrode placement should be made by a physician. The tip of the electrode is inserted at the spinous process. The electrode is then pushed deeper, down the side of the process until the tip is resting on the lamina. The exposed portion of the electrodes should then be protected from accidental movement.

There are advantages and disadvantages to both electrode placements. Percutaneous placement is technically difficult and can be dangerous. Stimulating electrodes frequently work their way out, requiring replacement during the surgical procedure, which is difficult to accomplish under sterile drapes. In contrast, the spinous process electrodes are placed by the surgeon with direct visualization of anatomic structures. Typically, replacement of spinous process electrodes is not necessary during the case.

There are problems with placement in the wound, the most common of which is moisture. Too much blood or irrigation fluid can cause spread or shunting of the current and, thus, decrease the stimulus intensity level reaching the spinal cord. This can be recognized by a decrease in evoked potential amplitude that improves following suctioning of fluid from the wound. Another problem area is the interface of electrode and bone, which must remain moist or impedance at the stimulus site will increase, resulting in less current reaching the spinal cord. This is recognized by increased stimulus artifact and should resolve by placing the electrodes in a different place within the spinous process.

A problem inherent to both stimulation methods is the requirement of adequate muscle relaxation to avoid patient movement on the operating table and contamination of response from myogenic activity. The anesthesiologist must titrate neuromuscular blocking agents in a dose adequate to eliminate patient movement.

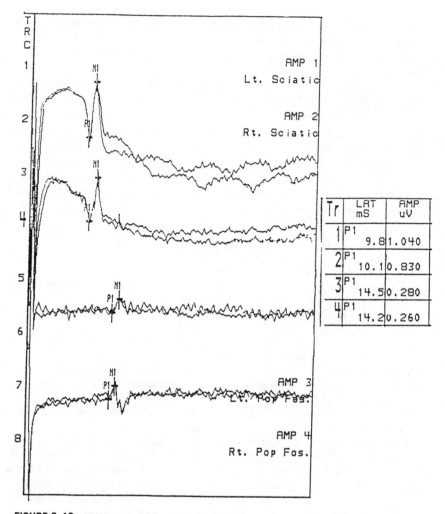

Tr	LAT mS	AMP uV
1	P1 9.8	1.040
2	P1 10.1	0.830
3	P1 14.5	0.280
4	P1 14.2	0.260

FIGURE 9-13. NMEPs recorded from the sciatic notch and the popliteal fossa.

Another problem is reduction in response amplitude following placement of instrumentation such as a rod or plate. This is typically a critical point in surgery when responses are observed closely to monitor for potential neural damage. Presence of the instrumentation itself can cause reduction in response amplitude. This is attributed to the stimulus current "jumping" the rod or plate, resulting in current spread. Increase of stimulus intensity should resolve response amplitude reduction. If not, stimulating electrodes should be placed further from the instrumentation. If responses fail to improve following these measures, surgical reasons for reduction in responses should be considered.

According to Owen (1991) a warning criteria of 60% reduction in amplitude is appropriate. However, intervention such as a Stagnara wake-up test is not employed unless response amplitude degrades further. in our experience of more than 1,000 spine cases in 5 years, damage to the motor pathways typically results in near or total obliteration of the NMEP response.

There is clear indication for use of NMEPs during surgical procedures in which the spinal cord is placed at risk. Used in conjunction with SEPs, valuable information concerning the sensory and motor tracts of the spinal cord is provided for the surgeon.

REFERENCES

Ben-David, B., Haller, G., & Taylor, P. (1987). Anterior spinal fusion complicated by paraplegia. *Spine, 12* (6), 536.

Bradshaw, K., Webb, J. K., & Fraser, A. M. (1984). Clinical evaluation of spinal cord monitoring in scoliosis surgery. *Spine, 9* (6), 636.

Chiappa, K., & Ropper, A. (1982). Evoked potentials in clinical medicine. *New England Journal of Medicine, 306,*(20), 1140–1150.

Cruse, R., Klem, G., Lesser, R. P., & Lueders, H. (1982). Paradoxical lateralization of cortical potentials evoked by stimulation of posterior tibial nerve. *Archives of Neurology, 39,* 222.

Harner, P. F., & Sannit, T. (1974). *A review of the international ten-twenty system of electrode placement.* Quincy, MA: Grass Instrument Company.

Hufnagel, A., Elger, C. E., Durwen, H. F., Boker, D.K.,& Entzian, W. (1989 August). *Activity of the epileptic focus by transcranial magnetic stimulation of the human brain.* Paper presented at the International motor evoked potential symposium, Chicago.

Jasper, H. H. (1958). Report of committee on methods of clinical examination in EEG. Appendix: The ten-twenty electrode system of the International Federation. *Electroencephalography and Clinical Neurophysiology, 10,* 371.

Jones, S. J., Howard, L., & Shawkat, F. (1988). Criteria for detection and pathological significance of response decrement during spinal cord monitoring. In T. Ducker & R. Brown (Eds.) *Neurophysiology and standards of spinal cord monitoring* (p. 201). New York: Springer-Verlag.

Keith, R. W., Stambough, J. L., & Awender, S. H. (1990). Somatosensory cortical evoked potentials: A review of 100 cases of intraoperative spinal surgery monitoring. *Journal of Spinal Disorders, 3* (3), 220.

Lesser, R. P., Raudzens, P., Lueders, H., Nuwer, M. R., Goldie, W. D., Morris, H. H., Dinner, D. S., Klem, G., Hahn, J. F., Shetter, A. G., Ginsburg, H. H., & Gurd, A. R. (1986). Postoperative neurological deficits may occur despite unchanged intraoperative somatosensory evoked potentials. *Annals of Neurology, 19* (1), 22.

Lesser, R. P., Stambough, J. L., Awender, S. H. (1981). Early somatosensory potentials evoked by median nerve stimulation: Intraoperative monitoring. *Neurology, 31,* 1519.

Machida, M., Asai, T., Sato, K., Toriyama, S., & Yamada, T. (1986). New approach for diagnosis in herniated lumbosacral disc: Dermatomal somatosensory evoked potentials. *Spine, 11* (4), 380.

Mustain, W., & Kendig, R. (1991). Dissociation of neurogenic motor and somatosensory evoked potentials. *Spine, 16* (7), 851.

Nielson, C. H. (1991). Anesthesia for spinal surgery. In K. Bridwell & R. Dewald (Eds.), *The textbook of spinal surgery* (pp. 19–31) Philadelphia: J. B. Lippincott.

Nuwer, M. R., & Dawson, E. C. (1984). Intraoperative evoked potential monitoring of the spinal cord. *Clinical Orthopedics, 183,* 42.

Obrien, M. F., Lenke, L. G., Padberg, A. M., Bridwell, K. H., & Stokes, R. M. (1993). *Evoked potential monitoring of the upper extremities during thoracic and lumbar spinal deformity surgery: A prospective study.* Paper presented at Scoliosis Research Society annual meeting, Dublin.

Owen, J. H., Laschinger, J.C., Bridwell, K. H., Shimon, S. M., & Nielsen, C.H. (1988). Sensitivity and specificity of somatosensory and neurogenic-motor evoked potentials in animals and humans. *Spine, 12,* 1111.

Owen, J. H., Padberg, A. M., Holland, L. S., Bridwell, K. H., Keppler, L., & Steffee, A. (1991). Clinical correlation between degenerative spine disease and dermatomal somatosensory evoked potentials in humans. *Spine, 16* (Suppl. 6), 201.

Owen, J. H. (1991). Evoked potential monitoring during spinal cord surgery. In K. Bridwell & R. Dewald (Eds.), *The textbook of spinal surgery* (pp. 31–66) Philadelphia: J. B. Lippincott.

Stedman's Medical Dictionary (25th ed.). (1990). Baltimore: Williams and Wilkins.

Tamaki, T., Takano, H., & Inoue, S. (1981). The prevention of iatrogenic spinal cord injury utilizing the evoked spinal cord potential. *International Orthopedics, 4,* 313.

RECOMMENDED READINGS

Abel, M. F., Mubavak, S. J., & Wenser, O. R. (1990). Brainstem evoked potentials for scoliosis surgery: A reliable method allowing use of halogenated anesthetic agents. *Journal of Pediatric Orthopedics, 10,* 208.

Ben-David, B. (1988). Spinal cord monitoring. *Orthopedic Clinics of North America, 19* (2), 427.

Bunch, W. H., Scharff, T. B., & Trimble, J. (1983). Spinal cord monitoring. *Journal of Bone and Joint Surgery, 65-A*(5), 707.

Dawson, G. D. (1947). Cerebral responses to electrical stimulation of peripheral nerve in man. *Journal of Neurology and Psychiatry, 10,* 137.

Eisen, A., & Elleker, G. (1979). Sensory nerve stimulation and evoked cerebral potentials. *Neurology, 30,* 1097.

Griffiths, I. R., Trench, J. G., & Crawford, R. A. (1979). Spinal cord blood flow and conduction during experimental cord compression in normotensive and hypotensive dogs. *Journal of Neurosurgery, 50,* 353.

Leuders, H., Dinner, D., Lesser, R., & Klem, G. (1987). Origin of far field subcortical evoked potentials to posterior tibial and median nerve stimulation. *Archives of Neurology, 40,* 93.

MacEwen, G. D., Bunnell, W. P., & Sriram, K. (1975). Acute neurological complications in treatment of scoliosis. *Journal of Bone and Joint Surgery, 57-A*(3), 404.

Nash, C. L., & Brown, R. H. (1979). The intraoperative monitoring of spinal cord function: Its growth and current status. *Orthopedic Clinics of North America, 10*(1), 919.

Owen, J. H., Naito, M., & Bridwell, K. H., (1990). Relationship between duration of lost evoked potentials and clinical status in animals. *Spine, 15,* 618.

Tolmie, J. D., & Birch, A. A. (1991). *Anesthesia for the uninterested.* Gaithersburg, MD: Aspen Publishers.

■ SECTION THREE ■

THE PHYSICIAN'S PERSPECTIVE

◼ CHAPTER 10 ◼

VESTIBULAR NERVE SECTION

◼ DERALD E. BRACKMANN, M.D. ◼

Vestibular nerve section is the most definitive method of controlling disabling vertigo in patients who have failed medical or more conservative surgical therapy. The most common indication for vestibular nerve section is disabling vertigo secondary to Meniere's disease. Other etiologies are posttraumatic vertigo, postsurgical vertigo, and persistent disabling symptoms following an episode of vestibular neuronitis.

There are three techniques that may be utilized to section the vestibular nerve. The approach depends on the residual hearing in the diseased ear and the surgeon's preference. Monitoring of the facial nerve is an integral part of each of these techniques.

Selective section of the vestibular nerve with preservation of hearing may be performed via the middle fossa or retrolabyrinthine routes. When hearing is not a consideration, total labyrinthectomy and section of the entire CN VIII is performed via a translabyrinthine approach.

Regardless of the approach, the facial nerve is in close proximity and, in some cases, actually adherent to the vestibular nerve. Facial nerve monitoring aids in the identification and prevention of injury to the facial nerve during the surgical procedure.

In addition to facial nerve monitoring, some surgeons have utilized either far field or direct CN VIII monitoring in selective vestibular nerve section. Far field auditory brainstem response (ABR) monitoring is not helpful in preservation of hearing, because the events recorded are delayed by several minutes. On the other hand, direct CN VIII recordings may provide real-time information and be helpful in preserving hearing.

The techniques for CN VII and CN VIII monitoring have been discussed previously. What follows are the indications, surgical techniques, results, and complications for each of the three methods of vestibular nerve section.

RETROLABYRINTHINE VESTIBULAR NERVE SECTION

INDICATIONS

Retrolabyrinthine vestibular nerve section is indicated for patients with disabling vertigo and normal or aidable hearing. These patients have failed medical treatment and, in most cases, an endolymphatic sac procedure. Occasionally, a retrolabyrinthine vestibular nerve section is performed as a primary procedure for patients with advanced Meniere's disease.

The retrolabyrinthine vestibular nerve section has low morbidity and is well tolerated by patients of all ages. A disadvantage of the procedure is that the lack of a clear cleavage plane between the cochlear and vestibular nerves may lead to incomplete nerve section in a small percentage of cases.

SURGICAL TECHNIQUES

The patient is prepared and draped for standard postauricular mastoidectomy. A large curvilinear incision is made approximately 2 cm behind the postauricular crease. The posterior position of this incision allows greater exposure of the sigmoid sinus, which aids in its decompression.

With use of an operating microscope and continuous suction irrigation, a complete, simple mastoidectomy is performed. The lateral and posterior semicircular canal is not blue-lined. Generally the incus is not exposed and it should not come into contact with the drill, as this could result in sensorineural hearing loss. The facial nerve is not routinely exposed.

Bone is removed from over the sigmoid sinus and the posterior fossa dura behind it is exposed. An island of bone (Bill's island) is usually left over the lateral surface of the sigmoid sinus to protect it. Wide sigmoid sinus decompression is the key to adequate exposure by this route. The middle fossa dura and posterior fossa dura are then skeletonized and all bone is removed from behind the labyrinth to the sigmoid sinus. Should bleeding occur from the superior petrosal sinus or mastoid emissary vein, it can be controlled by bipolar cautery, bone wax, or sutures. After complete skeletonization of the posterior fossa dura, a large, anteriorly based U-shaped dural flap is fashioned. The apex of the flap runs parallel to the sigmoid sinus and the endolymphatic sac is preserved. The dural flap is then reflected anteriorly and secured with a silk suture.

Large cottonoids are placed over the surface of the cerebellum and the cerebellopontine angle is entered. As spinal fluid is released, the cerebellum falls away, exposing the cranial nerves. Mannitol and Furosemide are used for dehydration of the brain to achieve greater exposure.

On entering the cerebellopontine angle, the surgeon identifies the cranial nerves. The CN V lies cephalad and is the largest. The CN IX lies caudad and is the smallest. The CN VII and CN VIII lie between these two. The facial nerve is directly anterior to the CN VIII and is usually hidden by it. Gentle retraction of the CN VIII enables identification of the facial nerve. The auditory and vestibular divisions of the CN VIII lie together at this point and must be separated (Figure 10-1). The vestibular portion makes up the cephalad half of the nerve. The vestibular nerve is more greyish in color than the white cochlear nerve. In many cases, no obvious demarcation exists. Occasionally, a small vessel will run along the division of the two nerves. The cephalad portion of the nerve is divided with a sharp hook or neurectomy scissors. Generally, when the division of the vestibular nerve is complete, the nerve stumps will retract.

Abdominal fat is harvested, cut into strips, and used to pack the mastoid cavity. The postauricular incision is closed in layers and a standard pressure dressing is placed on the wound. The patient is observed in the intensive care unit for 1 day postoperatively and usually hospitalized for 5 or 6 days.

RESULTS

The rate of control of vertigo by retrolabyrinthine vestibular nerve section ranges from 93 to 97% (Silverstein, McDaniel, Wazen & Norrell, 1985). This is comparable to reported results of middle fossa vestibular nerve section. Persistent postoperative unsteadiness does occur, but it is rarely considered disabling by the patient. Hearing is maintained near the preoperative level in 75 to 78% of the patients with retrolabyrinthine vestibular nerve section. Total hearing losses occur postoperatively in approximately 2% (McElveen, Shelton, Hitselberger, & Brackmann, 1988). Hearing results after retrolabyrinthine vestibular nerve section are reported to be superior to those after middle fossa vestibular nerve section (De la Cruz & McElveen, 1984).

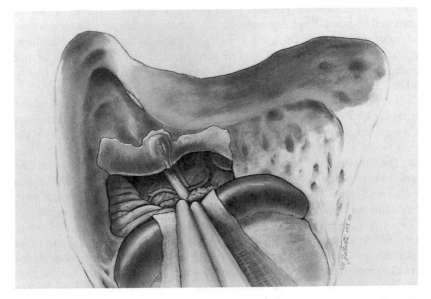

FIGURE 10–1. Retrolabyrinthine exposure of the right CN VIII with the facial nerve seen anteriorly. The vestibular fibers are sectioned in the superior half of the CN VIII.

The cause of postoperative hearing loss is unclear. It could possibly be related to cochlear nerve and labyrinthine artery trauma, transection of the endolymphatic duct, unrecognized fenestration of the posterior canal, or natural progression of the Meniere's disease. Some patients have postoperative conductive hearing loss. This may be due to ossicular fixation from bone dust produced during the mastoidectomy or impingement of abdominal fat on the ossicular heads. To prevent this complication, we do not routinely expose the ossicular heads during the mastoid dissection and we thoroughly irrigate the mastoid antrum after drilling.

Silverstein et al. (1985) advocate intraoperative auditory brainstem response (ABR) and direct CN VIII monitoring during nerve section. We routinely monitor our cases in this fashion. Although intraoperative ABR has not been helpful in our experience, direct CN VIII monitoring does give some useful information.

COMPLICATIONS

Facial nerve paralysis is a theoretical postoperative complication, but has not occurred in any of our more than 600 cases. Cerebrospinal fluid (CSF) leaks have occurred in approximately 5%. Most cases of CSF leaks respond to a mastoid pressure dressing and/or lumbar drainage. Rarely is it necessary to re-explore the wound and add more abdominal fat. Meningitis is an infrequent complication in our series.

DISCUSSION

Selective vestibular nerve section by the suboccipital route was first reported by McKenzie in 1936. Previously, total CN VIII section for the treatment of Meniere's disease was reported by Frazier (1912), Cairns and Brain (1933), and Dandy (1928). These early authors noted that many patients, even those after total CN VIII section and resulting total sensorineural hearing loss, had persistent tinnitus.

The retrolabyrinthine approach has been used for many years for access to the cerebellopontine angle. Brackmann and Hitselberger (1978) employed this route for access to the trigeminal nerve and for biopsy of tumors in the cerebellopontine angle. This approach for vestibular nerve section was popularized by Silverstein and Norrell (1980). In the retrolabyrinthine approach, there may not be an evident cleavage plane between the vestibular and cochlear nerves. There appears to be intermingling of vestibular and cochlear fibres in the region between the two nerves (Natout, Terr, Linthicum, & House, 1987).

The retrosigmoid approach to the internal auditory meatus has been advocated as an alternative to the retrolabyrinthine route. Access to the CN VIII at a location with a clear cleavage plane is provided by the retrosigmoid approach (Millen & Meyer, 1986; Silverstein, Norrell, & Smouha, 1987). However, severe postoperative headaches after retrosigmoid craniotomy are seen in a substantial number of patients. Silverstein (personal communication) has recently introduced a new modification, a combined retrolabyrinthine/retrosigmoid approach. It combines the advantages of both approaches, but has a lower incidence of postoperative headache.

When a selective vestibular nerve section is indicated, we prefer the retrolabyrinthine over the middle fossa approach. It is better tolerated by older patients because it avoids temporal lobe retraction. Dissection is technically easier and exposure is wider. In our experience, the two approaches produce comparable results for control of vertigo and hearing preservation.

MIDDLE FOSSA VESTIBULAR NERVE SECTION

INDICATIONS

The middle fossa approach provides access to the vestibular nerve as a discrete entity separate from the cochlear nerve. The indications for the middle fossa vestibular nerve section are the same as for retrolabyrinthine nerve section. The middle fossa approach is generally reserved for younger patients, because the middle fossa dura is more difficult to elevate in an older patient and the elderly tolerate temporal lobe retraction less well. At the House Ear Clinic (HEC), we perform most vestibular nerve sections by the retrolabyrinthine approach and reserve the middle fossa approach for revision of the rare retrolabyrinthine vestibular nerve section failure.

SURGICAL TECHNIQUE

The patient is placed on the table in the supine position with the head turned to the side and the surgeon is seated at the head of the table. A curvilinear incision approximately 6 to 7 cm long starts anterior to the tragus and proceeds superiorly, curving slightly posteriorly.

The temporalis muscle is divided in a U-shaped flap based inferiorly at the zygomatic arch. The temporalis muscle flap is reflected inferiorly and the squamous portion of the temporal bone is exposed with a self-retaining retractor.

A craniotomy measuring 5 cm square is made in the squamous portion of the temporal bone. Two-thirds of the opening is located anterior to the external auditory meatus; one-third is located posteriorly. A medium-sized cutting burr is used to outline the craniotomy window. Care should be taken not to lacerate the dura during this bone removal to prevent herniation of the temporal lobe. The dura is separated from the edges of the craniotomy defect and the House-Urban middle fossa retractor is then inserted. The arms of the self-retaining retractors are locked against the bony margins of the craniotomy defect. As the middle fossa dura is elevated, the retractor blade is advanced. The anterior limit of the dural elevation is the middle meningeal artery exiting the foramen spinosum. Bleeding may be encountered from the foramen. This bleeding usually originates from venous channels and is easily controlled with Surgicel packing. The middle fossa dura is then elevated in a posterior-to-anterior direction to prevent injury to the facial nerve. The posterior-to-anterior dissection prevents elevation of the greater superficial petrosal nerve and avoids injury to the geniculate ganglion. In some patients, the arcuate eminence may be an obvious landmark, but this is not consistently encountered. The greater superficial petrosal nerve is then identified and followed posteriorly to the geniculate ganglion.

With the greater superficial petrosal nerve as a landmark, bone is removed over the area of the geniculate ganglion and it is identified. Continuous suction irrigation and a large diamond burr are used for this bone removal. Injury to the geniculate ganglion is avoided by leaving a thin eggshell of bone over it.

The facial nerve is followed through its labyrinthine portion to the internal auditory meatus. Care is taken to avoid the cochlea, which lies directly anteriorly. The ampulla of the superior semicircular canal is several millimeters posterior to the facial nerve. The superior semicircular canal makes an angle of 45° to 60° with the internal auditory meatus.

The superior surface of the internal auditory meatus is skeletonized, avoiding injury to the dura. Dissection of the lateral end of the internal auditory meatus reveals the vertical crest of bone (Bill's bar) that separates the superior vestibular nerve from the facial nerve.

The dura of the internal auditory meatus is opened at a point distant from the facial nerve. The superior vestibular nerve is identified in the posterior superior aspect of the internal auditory meatus. It is separated from the facial nerve and divided medial to Scarpa's ganglion. The inferior vestibular nerve is identified deeper in the meatus and also sectioned medial to Scarpa's ganglion (Figure 10–2). Bipolar cautery is used to achieve hemostasis and a free graft of temporalis muscle is used to plug the internal auditory meatus defect. The temporal lobe is allowed to expand and the craniotomy bone flap is replaced. The wound is closed in layers, usually with

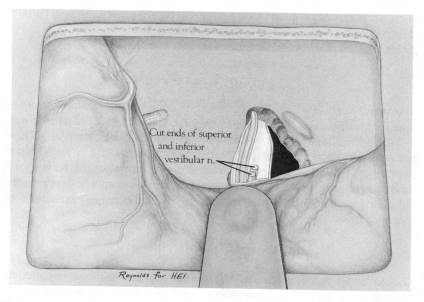

Cut ends of superior
and inferior
vestibular n.

Reynolds for HEI

FIGURE 10–2. Middle fossa exposure of the right internal auditory meatus with preganglionic section of the vestibular nerves.

placement of a Penrose drain. A sterile pressure dressing is applied and remains for approximately 4 days. Postoperatively, the patient is observed in the intensive care unit for 24 hours. The patient is ambulatory the second postoperative day and remains hospitalized for 4 to 5 days postoperatively.

RESULTS

Glasscock, Kveton, and Christiansen (1984) reported control of vertigo in 94% of cases of middle fossa vestibular nerve section. Glasscock feels that patients over 60 years old have an increased risk of intracranial complications by this approach because the dura is thinner, bleeds excessively, and is easily torn.

Fisch (1984), reports similar rate of control of vertigo in Meniere's patients with a modified middle fossa approach for vestibular nerve section. His modification results in less temporal lobe retraction and, he feels, fewer complications. He prefers the middle fossa approach over the "less effective" retrolabyrinthine approach.

Hearing is stabilized or improved in 51 to 83% of patients undergoing middle fossa vestibular nerve section. The basis for this improvement is unclear, but may be related to section of the vestibulofacial anastomoses and resultant lysis of parasympathetic function to the cochlea (Garcia-Ibanez & Garcia-Ibanez, 1980). Improvement of tinnitus after middle fossa vestibular nerve section is unpredictable and occurs in approximately 50% of patients (Fisch, 1984; Garcia-Ibanez & Garcia-Ibanez, 1980; Gavilan & Gavilan, 1984; Glasscock, Hughes, Davis, & Jackson, 1980).

COMPLICATIONS

Transient facial nerve paralysis is the most common complication occurring after middle fossa vestibular nerve section. It occurs in 3 to 7% of cases (Fisch, 1984; Garcia-Ibanez & Garcia-Ibanez, 1980; Glasscock et al., 1980). These results were reported before the routine use of intraoperative facial nerve monitoring. Facial nerve paresis is much less common when this technique is used. In approximately 5% of cases, total hearing loss occurs postoperatively. Subdural hematoma, CSF leak, and meningitis each occur in less than 2% of cases.

DISCUSSION

Middle fossa CN VIII section for the treatment of dizziness was reported by Parry in 1904. This approach was fully developed in 1961 by William House who used it for selective section of the vestibular nerve. The middle fossa approach has the advantage of an extradural dissection and allows access to the complete contents of the internal auditory meatus. This exposure allows section of the vestibular nerves as anatomically separate entities from the cochlear nerve.

The middle fossa approach is more technically demanding. It has fewer landmarks than the retrolabyrinthine approach and is generally a bloodier procedure. I now perform vestibular nerve sections by the retrolabyrinthine approach and reserve the middle fossa approach for the rare retrolabyrinthine failure. In these revision cases, the complete exposure of the internal auditory canal assures total section of all remaining vestibular nerve fibers.

TRANSLABYRINTHINE VESTIBULAR NERVE SECTION

INDICATIONS

The gold standard for control of vertigo is the translabyrinthine vestibular nerve section. It allows removal of all neuroepithelium under direct vision and enables the surgeon to perform a preganglionic section of the vestibular nerves. We reserve this operation for patients with disabling vertigo and nonaidable hearing.

SURGICAL TECHNIQUE

The patient is prepared and draped for standard mastoid surgery. A postauricular incision is made approximately 2 cm behind the postauricular crease and the mastoid cortex is exposed with self-retaining retractor insertion.

A complete simple mastoidectomy is performed with continuous suction irrigation and a large cutting burr. The mastoid antrum is entered and the lateral semicircular canal is identified. The tegmen and sigmoid sinus are skeletonized. In a contracted mastoid, it may be necessary to decompress the sigmoid sinus (described in the section under retrolabyrinthine nerve section) for better exposure.

The labyrinthectomy is performed in a superior-to-inferior direction with the side of the cutting burr. The initial bone removal is in the supralabyrinthine air cell tract in the sinodural angle along the superior petrosal sinus. This opening is then widened progressively using the side of the cutting burr to remove the labyrinthine bone. Each semicircular canal is removed in a systematic fashion and used as a landmark for identification of the other canals. The lateral semicircular canal is opened and the common crus identified. The superior semicircular canal is removed; its ampulla is saved as a landmark for the superior vestibular nerve. The vestibule is opened and will serve as a landmark for the lateral end of the internal auditory meatus.

It is important to skeletonize the facial nerve to allow adequate visualization of the vestibule and lateral end of the internal auditory meatus. This is accomplished with the side of a diamond burr. Because the labyrinthine bone has been previously removed, the plane between the burr and the facial nerve may be directly viewed at all times. Adequate skeletonization of the nerve greatly enhances exposure of the lateral internal auditory meatus.

The internal auditory meatus is dissected. The dura of the internal auditory canal is skeletonized leaving a thin eggshell of bone over it. The dissection starts along the superior petrosal sinus and proceeds inferiorly to remove the retrofacial air cells and identify the jugular bulb.

The internal auditory meatus is skeletonized for approximately 180° of its circumference and three-quarters of its length. In contrast to the exposure needed for acoustic tumor removal, bone over the porus acousticus may be preserved. Inferior to the auditory meatus, the cochlea aqueduct may be encountered. Dissection should not proceed beyond this point to avoid injury to the lower cranial nerves.

The lateral end of the internal auditory meatus is dissected with identification of the singular and inferior vestibular nerves. The transverse crest is identified next. Superior to it lies the superior vestibular nerve. Directly anterior to the superior vestibular nerve, the facial nerve is identified with the bar of bone (Bill's bar) that separates the two (Figure 10–3). The thin shell of bone overlying the dura of the internal auditory meatus is now picked away. A small hook is passed on the posterior surface of Bill's bar and used to remove the superior vestibular nerve from the lateral end of the internal auditory meatus. The dura of the internal auditory meatus is then incised with fine scissors and the vestibular facial anastomosis is lysed with a fine hook. The inferior vestibular nerve is identified and retracted posteriorly. Scarpa's ganglia are identified by the enlargement of the nerves at that point. Fine neurectomy scissors are used to divide the nerve medial to Scarpa's ganglia, which are removed.

Abdominal fat is harvested and cut into strips, which are used to obliterate the mastoid cavity and the dural defect. The postauricular incision is closed in layers and a standard mastoid dressing is applied.

RESULTS

Control of vertigo after translabyrinthine vestibular nerve section has been reported to range from 93 to 98% (Nelson, 1986; Pulec, 1974). A few patients have postural unsteadiness postoperatively. This unsteadiness results from poor central compensation and is more prominent in older patients.

All patients experience a total neurosensory hearing loss after translabyrinthine vestibular nerve section. If tinnitus is a prominent symptom, I also

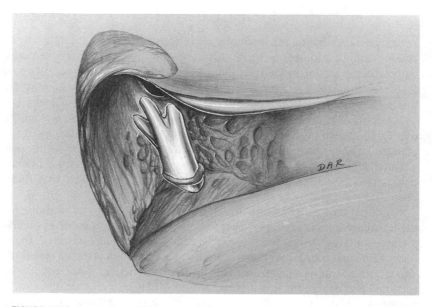

FIGURE 10–3. Translabyrinthine exposure of the right internal auditory meatus. The facial nerve is located anteriorosuperiorly and is separated from the superior vestibular nerve by Bill's bar. The transverse crest separates the superior and inferior vestibular nerves.

section the cochlear nerve during this procedure. Otherwise it is saved. The cochlear implant has been successfully used after translabyrinthine vestibular nerve section. Preservation of the cochlear nerve will preserve potential implant use if an unforeseen hearing loss occurs in the opposite ear.

COMPLICATIONS

Nelson found that 8% of 203 patients who had translabyrinthine vestibular nerve sections suffered transient facial palsy (Nelson, 1982). This was prior to the use of intraoperative monitoring and is much reduced using the technique. Paresis may develop after exposure of the facial nerve during the labyrinthectomy or because of lysis of adhesions between the facial and superior vestibular nerve at the lateral end of the internal auditory meatus. CSF leaks occurred in 6% and meningitis in 2% of the 203 patients studied by Nelson. My present routine procedure of packing the mastoid defect with abdominal fat before closure has reduced the incidence of CSF leaks and meningitis.

DISCUSSION

Although translabyrinthine vestibular nerve section is the most certain way to ablate vestibular function, some advocate transmastoid labyrinthectomy without nerve section instead (Graham & Kemink, 1984; Benecke, Tubegen, & Miyamoto, 1986). They feel that intracranial complications may be minimized by avoiding violation of the subarachnoid space.

Schuknecht (1982) feels that vestibular nerve section has no advantage over labyrinthectomy alone. He cites animal work that shows atrophy of the afferent vestibular neurons after transtympanic labyrinthectomy. Although acknowledging that traumatic vestibular neuromas have been seen in human temporal bones after postganglionic nerve section, he doubts that these neuromas can actually cause vestibular symptoms.

For patients with no useful hearing and disabling vertigo, I recommend the translabyrinthine vestibular nerve section. Because it provides a preganglionic section of the vestibular nerves, I prefer it to transmastoid labyrinthectomy. I feel that translabyrinthine vestibular nerve section is the most certain way to ablate labyrinthine function. In my experience, vestibular nerve section does not significantly increase the morbidity of the procedure over a transmastoid labyrinthectomy and the added assurance of the nerve section is worth the theoretical increased risk of an intracranial procedure.

CONCLUSION

Selective or total section of the vestibular nerve is an effective means of controlling disabling vertigo when more conservative measures have failed. These are well tolerated procedures with minimum morbidity and virtually no mortality. Intraoperative monitoring of the CN VII and CN VIII adds significantly to the safety of these procedures.

REFERENCES

Benecke, J. E. Jr., Tubergen, L. B., Miyamoto, R. T. (1986). Transmastoid labyrintectomy. *American Journal of Otology, 7,* 41-43.

Brackmann, D. E., & Hitselberger, W. E., (1978). Retrolabyrinthine approach: Technique and newer indications. *Laryngoscope, 88,* 286-297.

Cairns, H., & Brain, W. R. (1933). Aural vertigo: Treatment by division of the eighth nerve. *Lancet, 1* (5723), 946-952.

Dandy, W. E., (1928). Meniere's disease: Its diagnosis and a method of treatment. *Archives of Surgery, 16,* 1127-1152.

De la Cruz, A., McElveen, J. T. (1984). Hearing preservation in vestibular neurectomy. *Laryngoscope, 94,* 874-877.

Fisch, U. (1984). Vestibular nerve section for Meniere's disease. *American Journal of Otology, 5,* 543–545.

Frazier, C. H. (1912). Intracranial division of the auditory nerve for persistent aural vertigo. *Surgery, Gynecology and Obstetrics, 15,* 524–529.

Garcia-Ibanez, E., & Garcia-Ibanez, J. L. (1980). Middle fossa vestibular neurectomy: A report of 373 cases. *Otolaryngology—Head and Neck Surgery, 88,* 486–190.

Gavilan, J., & Gavila, C. (1984). Middle fossa vestibular neurectomy. *Archives of Otolaryngology, 110,* 785–787.

Glasscock, M. E., Hughes, G. B., Davis, W. E., & Jackson, C. G. (1980). Labyrinthectomy versus middle fossa vestibular nerve section in Meniere's disease. *Annals of Otology, Rhinology and Laryngology, 89,* 318–324.

Glasscock, M. E., Kveton, J. F., & Christiansen, S. G. (1984). Middle fossa vestibular neurectomy: An update. *Otolaryngology—Head and Neck Surgery, 92,* 216–220.

Graham, M. D., & Kemink, J. L. (1984). Transmastoid labyrinthectomy: Surgical management of vertigo in the nonserviceable hearing ear. *American Journal of Otology, 5,* 295–299.

House, W. F. (1961). Surgical exposure of the internal auditory canal and its contents through the middle cranial fossa. *Laryngoscope, 71,* 1363–1385.

McElveen, J. T., Shelton, C., Hitselberger, W. E., & Brackmann, D. E. (1988). Retrolabyrinthine vestibular neurectomy: A re-evaluation. *Laryngoscope, 98,* 502–506.

McKenzie, K. G. (1936). Intracranial division of the vestibular portion of the auditory nerve for Meniere's disease. *Canadian Medical Association Journal, 34,* 369–381.

Millen, S. J., & Meyer, G. (1986). Retrosigmoid intracanalicular vestibular nerve section: An alternative surgical approach for Meniere's disease. *American Journal of Otology, 7,* 330–332.

Natout, M. A. Y., Terr, L. I., Linthicum, F. H., & House, W. F. (1987). Topography of vestibulocochlear nerve fibers in the posterior cranial fossa. *Laryngoscope 97,* 954–958.

Nelson, R. A. (1982). Labryrinthectomy and translabyrinthine nerve section. In Brackmann, D. E. (Ed.), *Neurological survey of the ear and skull base* (pp. 149–159). Philadelphia: B. C. Decker Inc.

Nelson, R. A. (1986). Surgery for control of vertigo. In R. J. Wiet & J. B. Causse (Eds.), *Complications in Otolaryngology—Head and neck surgery: Vol I: Ear and skull base* (pp. 149–159). Philadelphia: BC Decker Inc.

Parry, R. H. (1904). A case of tinnitus and vertigo treated by division of the auditory nerve. *Journal of Laryngology, Rhinology and Otology. 19,* 402–406.

Pulec, J. L. (1974). Labyrinthectomy: Indications, technique and results. *Laryngoscope, 84,* 1552–1573.

Schuknecht, H. F. (1982). Behavior of the vestibular nerve following labyrinthectomy. *Annals of Otology, Rhinology, and Laryngology, 91*(Suppl. 97), 16–32.

Silverstein, H., McDaniel, A., Wazen, J., & Norrell, H. (1985). Retrolabyrinthine vestibular neurectomy with simultaneous monitoring of eighth nerve and brain stem auditory evoked potentials. *Otolaryngology—Head and Neck Surgery, 93,* 7836–742.

Silverstein, H., & Norrell, H. (1980). Retrolabyrinthine surgery: A direct approach to the cerebellopontine angle. *Otolaryngology—Head and Neck Surgery, 88,* 462–469.

Silverstein, H., Norrell, H., & Smouha, E. E. (1987). Retrosigmoid-internal auditory canal approach vs. retrolabyrinthine approach for vestibulary neurectomy. *Otolaryngology—Head and Neck Surgery, 97,* 300–307.

■ CHAPTER 11 ■

ACOUSTIC NEUROMA SURGERY

■ ERIC W. SARGENT, M.D. ■

Acoustic neuromas are the third most common type of intracranial tumor, accounting for 8–10% of all intracranial tumors and about 75% of all tumors occurring in the *cerebellopontine angle* (CPA) (the area between the pons and cerebellum in the posterior fossa through which CN VII and VIII pass). The insidious progression of cranial nerve symptoms and intracranial hypertension culminating in death in patients with untreated acoustic tumors was described by Leveque-Lasource (1810) and Bell (1833) in the early nineteenth century.

Although a neuroma confined to the internal auditory canal (IAC) was noted by Toynbee in 1853, Henschen in 1915 first suggested that acoustic neuromas originate within the IAC and only secondarily extend into the CPA. It is now believed that most acoustic neuromas start in an area of the vestibular nerve rich in Schwann cells termed the *Obersteiner-Redlich zone* (Sterkers, Perre, Viala, & Foncin, 1987). Following the path of least resistance, the tumor extends from the IAC into the CPA. As the tumors typically originate from the Schwann cells (not neurons) that sheathe the fibers of the vestibular nerve (not the auditory nerve), they are more correctly termed *vestibular schwannomas;* however, because these lesions are most often called acoustic neuromas in the literature, they will be referred to as such throughout this chapter for the sake of uniformity.

Unilateral hearing loss and unilateral tinnitus have long been recognized as early symptoms of an acoustic neuroma (Cushing, 1932). When confined to the internal auditory canal (intracanalicular), the symptoms of an acoustic neuroma are typically hearing loss, tinnitus, and vertigo. In the cistern of the CPA, the patient may have no additional symptoms or may present with headache and disequilibrium, instead of vertigo.

Undiagnosed, the tumor may cause complete sensorineural hearing loss, compromise facial nerve function and sensation and may extend to and compress the brainstem—finally causing hydrocephalus and death.

The growth rate of these tumors is generally slow, but can vary widely. Wazen observed a yearly growth rate of 2 mm per year, but found a few tumors that grew up to 10 mm per year (Wazen, Silverstein, Norrell, & Besse, 1985). Because of their unpredictable growth and life-threatening potential, excision of acoustic neuromas is usually the treatment of choice. However, elderly asymptomatic patients and patients who are poor surgical candidates may elect to be followed with serial imaging studies.

Early diagnosis and treatment of acoustic neuromas are the keys to successful management. When these tumors are identified early and small, many options are available. When diagnosed as large lesions, surgical excision tends to be more difficult with increased risk of functional compromise.

The first successful excision of an acoustic neuroma was by Sir Charles Ballance (1907) in 1894. To a modern reader, the bravery of the patient and surgeon in an era when anesthetic was delivered by an ether cone, electrosurgical cautery had not been invented, and antibiotics had not been discovered is astounding. Between 1894 and 1910, the surgical mortality rate of acoustic neuroma resection was approximately 80%. Increased knowledge of vascular anatomy and improvement in anesthetics, plus patient monitoring and surgical instrumentation has decreased the operative mortality to 0.8–5%.

Preservation of facial nerve function was given low priority by early surgeons and postoperative facial nerve weakness was a uniform complication. Dandy (1941) stated "loss of the facial nerve is a small price to pay for the cure of an acoustic tumor." Patients frequently presented with a facial nerve palsy at diagnosis due to the delay in diagnosis caused by the lack of reliable diagnostic tests (Cross, 1981). Similarly, as preoperative hearing was uniformly poor, preservation of the auditory nerve was not considered (Cushing, 1932). Today, facial symptoms accompanying acoustic neuroma diagnosis are rare, as these tumors are often diagnosed while relatively small.

The problem is that as the acoustic neuroma grows, it progressively attenuates the auditory and facial nerves (Figure 11-1, bottom). In large tumors, the nerves may be reduced to a thin layer along the capsule of the tumor. The tumor may insinuate itself into the substance of the nerves, making dissection without significant manipulation impossible. Although

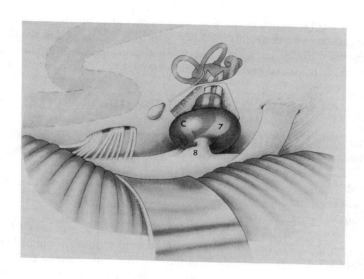

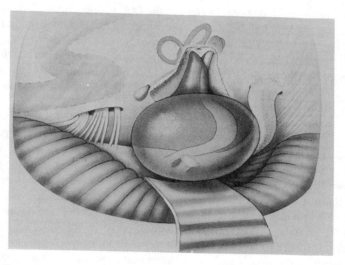

FIGURE 11–1. Top. Suboccipital view of a small left-sided acoustic neuroma. Note that the posterior lip of the internal auditory canal has been drilled away, exposing the tumor without entering the labyrinth. **Bottom.** A large left-sided acoustic neuroma that penetrates the internal auditory canal deeply, requiring exenteration of the labyrinth for exposure of the lateral extent of tumor. Note the marked splaying of the facial nerve over the posterior surface of the tumor. (From "Selection of surgical approach to acoustic neuroma" by R. W. Jackler, 1992, *Otolaryngologic Clinics of North America, 25,* p. 367. Copyright 1992 by W. B. Saunders Co. Reprinted by permission.)

hearing and facial nerve sacrifice was considered inevitable in the past, the introduction of the dissecting microscope in 1921 by Carl Nylen and the more recent use of facial and auditory nerve monitoring has made anatomical and oftentimes functional preservation of the nerves achievable.

SURGICAL APPROACHES: SUBOCCIPITAL

First described in 1904 by Fraenkel, Hunt, Woolsey, and Elsberg, the suboccipital approach was, and in some areas remains, the standard approach to the CPA.

Traditionally, the suboccipital approach was performed with the patient seated. Through a vertical incision extending well into the neck, a large segment of occipital bone was removed. In the past, a portion of the lateral cerebellum was removed, particularly in large tumors.

The suboccipital approach is used to remove tumors in the CPA of any size from the CPA, but cannot by itself be used to remove tumor from the lateral IAC. To remove tumor from the IAC, the bone must be drilled away or dissection is done blindly, jeopardizing the facial and cochlear nerves. In many instances, if the lateral extent of the IAC is fully exposed, the posterior semicircular canal will be opened, sacrificing hearing. The surgeon does not enter the otic capsule in the standard suboccipital procedure. This approach can be used in cases in which an attempt is made to preserve hearing if the tumor primarily resides in the CPA and has only minimal IAC extension.

The chief advantage of the suboccipital approach is the wide exposure of the tumor and relative ease of excision.

Weaknesses of the suboccipital operation include possible embolization of air sucked into open veins or dural venous sinuses when the patient is seated. This can be largely resolved by placing the patient supine with the head turned away from the surgeon or in the three-quarter prone position (Figure 11–2A). Resection of the lateral cerebellum leads to movement and coordination disorders that may be subtle or gross. Chronic postoperative neck pain and headache is common because of the dissection of the muscles from the skull base. This procedure is hampered by the blind approach the surgeon is forced to take with respect to the facial nerve. As the facial nerve is anterior to the tumor and the suboccipital approach is from posterior to anterior, the nerve cannot be visualized before it is put at-risk by dissection.

Table 11–1 summarizes the advantages and disadvantages of the traditional suboccipital approach.

RETROSIGMOID-TRANSMEATAL APPROACH

In 1973, Smith, Miller, and Cox described the results of a *neurotologic* retrosigmoid approach. In Smith's series, total tumor removal was performed in 14

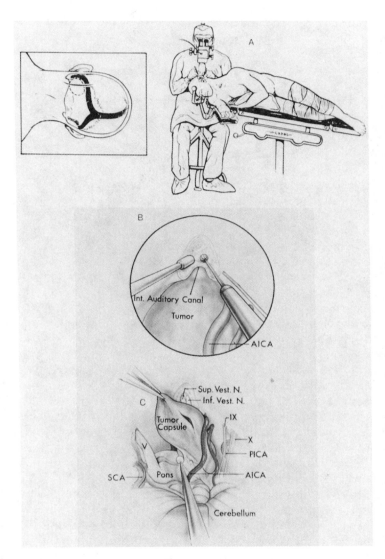

FIGURE 11-2A. Retrosigmoid approach to CPA, right ear. **(A)** Patient positioned in three-quarter prone position, incision with exposure of dura, sigmoid sinus, and cerebellum. **(B)** Drilling away the posterior wall of the internal auditory canal (AICA: anterior inferior cerebellar artery). **(C)** After removal of the contents of the acoustic neuroma, the capsule is removed from the pons. (From "Microsurgical Anatomy of Acoustic Neuroma" by A. L. Rhoton, Jr., and H. Tedeschi, 1992, *Otolaryngologic Clinics of North America, 25*, pp. 292-293. Copyright 1992 by W. B. Saunders Co. Reprinted by permission.)

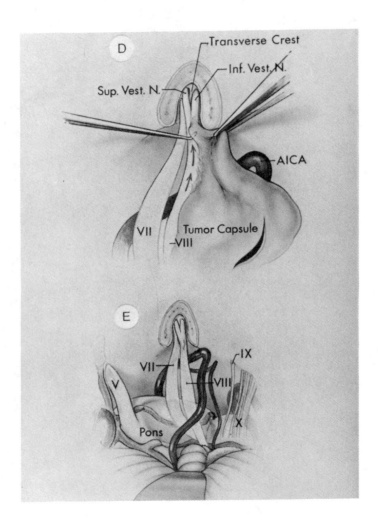

FIGURE 11-2B. *(Continued.)* Retrosigmoid approach to CPA, right ear. **(D)** In a hearing preservation procedure, dissection is performed from medial to lateral to prevent injury to the cochlear nerve as it inserts into the lamina cribrosa. **(E)** The CPA following tumor removal. (From "Microsurgical Anatomy of Acoustic Neuroma" by A. L. Rhoton, Jr., and H. Tedeschi, 1992, *Otolaryngologic Clinics of North America, 25,* pp. 292-293. Copyright 1992 by W. B. Saunders Co. Reprinted by permission.

of 15 patients. Postoperative facial function was normal in one small and six medium-sized tumors and "satisfactory" in five of eight large tumors. The remaining three of eight large tumors had total facial paralysis. This approach is often described as the retrosigmoid-transmeatal operation (Cohen, Hammerschlag, Berg, & Ransohoff, 1986; Giannotta & Pulec, 1988).

The CPA is approached through a small craniotomy situated directly behind the sigmoid sinus (Figure 11-2A). The incision does not extend into the neck and dissection of muscles from the skull base is minimized. The cerebellum is retracted posteriorly instead of resected. The lateral extent of the tumor is removed from the IAC by the neurotologist after the neurosurgeon debulks the mass of the tumor and dissects it from the brainstem.

The retrosigmoid-transmeatal approach can be used to remove tumors of any size from the CPA. This approach is often used when the surgeon is attempting to preserve hearing. (See Table 11-2.)

Strengths of the approach include less operative morbidity, as resection of the cerebellum is seldom necessary. However, retraction of the cerebellum required to expose larger tumors can itself lead to cerebellar atrophy and

TABLE 11-1. SUMMARY OF ADVANTAGES AND DISADVANTAGES OF THE SUBOCCIPITAL APPROACH.

Suboccipital Approach	
Advantages	*Disadvantages*
Wide exposure	Possible air embolus
Hearing preservation possible	Damage to cerebellum
	Chronic postop pain
	Blind approach to VII

TABLE 11-2. SUMMARY OF ADVANTAGES AND DISADVANTAGES OF THE RETROSIGMOID APPROACH.

Retrosigmoid Approach	
Advantages	*Disadvantages*
Good exposure	Blind approach to VII
Possible hearing preservation	
Less risk to cerebellum	

long-term coordination difficulties. The incidence of chronic postoperative headache is reduced due the decreased dissection of the muscles from the skull base. With the addition of the exposure of the contents of the IAC, the risk of recurrence from unresected tumor in the lateral IAC is reduced.

MIDDLE CRANIAL FOSSA APPROACH

In 1961 and 1962, William House presented the results of his approach to the IAC through the middle cranial fossa. Although originally designed to treat cochlear otosclerosis, this indication was eventually abandoned. However, the possibility of approaching lesions of the IAC through this approach was recognized.

The middle cranial fossa approach is indicated for the removal of small tumors confined to the IAC in patients with "good" preoperative hearing. Tumors that extend more than 5 mm beyond the porus acousticus are generally not removed by this approach. The definition of preoperative hearing sufficient to warrant the approach varies between different surgeons. Shelton, Brackmann, House, and Hitselberger (1989a) use a speech reception threshold of better than 30 dB and a speech discrimination score better than 70% as their criteria. Gantz, Parnes, Harker, and McCabe (1986) advocate an attempt at hearing conservation for patients with any measurable preoperative hearing.

The patient is positioned supine on the operating table with the operated ear upward. An S-shaped incision is made extending onto the scalp from anterior to the ear. The temporalis muscle is incised along the superior temporal line, leaving a cuff of temporalis fascia to which the muscle can be sewn at the end of the procedure. This is done to maintain as much muscle as possible in case facial reanimation with temporalis muscle is required later. The muscle is reflected inferiorly. A 2.5–3 cm square bone flap, centered over the root of the zygomatic bone and external auditory canal, is raised (Figure 11–3A).

A self-retaining retractor with an independent middle arm (House-Urban or similar retractor) is secured to the edges of the craniotomy. The dura of the temporal lobe is elevated from the floor of the middle cranial fossa (Figure 11–3B). The middle arm of the retractor is incrementally advanced. The dissection is limited anteriorly and medially by the middle meningeal artery and posteriorly by the superior petrosal sinus at the petrous ridge. Elevation of the dura of the temporal lobe proceeds from posterior to anterior to minimize the chance of injury to the geniculate ganglion. Approximately 15% of patients demonstrate a dehiscent facial nerve at this location (Rhoton, Pulec, & Hall, 1968). The *arcuate eminence*, traditionally used to locate the

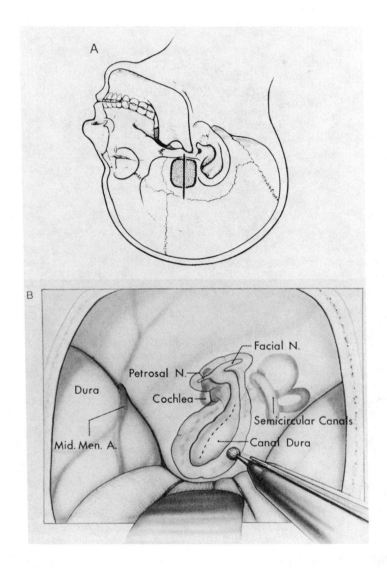

FIGURE 11–3A. Middle cranial fossa approach, right ear **(A)** Site of craniotomy. **(B)** Drilling the floor of the middle cranial fossa to expose the internal auditory canal following elevation of the dura. (From "Microsurgical Anatomy of Acoustic Neuroma" by A. L. Rhoton, Jr., and H. Tedeschi, 1992, *Otolaryngologic Clinics of North America*, 25, pp. 289-290. Copyright 1992 by W. B. Saunders Co. Reprinted by permission.)

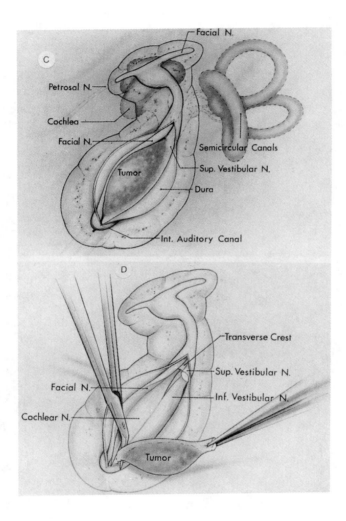

FIGURE 11–3B. Middle cranial fossa approach, right ear **(C)** The contents of the internal auditory canal following incision of the dura. **(D)** Removal of the tumor from the internal auditory canal after it has been separated from the facial and cochlear nerves. (From "Microsurgical Anatomy of Acoustic Neuroma" by A. L. Rhoton, Jr., and H. Tedeschi, 1992, *Otolaryngologic Clinics of North America*, 25, pp. 289-290. Copyright 1992 by W. B. Saunders Co. Reprinted by permission.)

position of the superior semicircular canal, is on the floor of the middle cranial fossa. Although absent in 15% of patients, the lateral aspect of the arcuate eminence predicts the location of the lateral limb of the superior semicircular canal in 98% of patients (Kartush, Kemink, & Graham, 1985).

The facial nerve is located using a number of different methods, the choice depending on the surgeon's experience and training. One method involves exposing the superior semicircular canal without entering it ("blue-lining"), then following the canal anteriorly to identify the facial nerve. A second method involves finding the greater superficial petrosal nerve anteriorly on the floor of the middle cranial fossa and following it posteriorly to the geniculate ganglion.

Surgical tolerances are extraordinarily limited in the area of the lateral IAC. Immediately posterior to the lateral IAC is the ampulated end of the superior semicircular canal; anteriorly, separated by millimeters from the labyrinthine segment of the facial nerve, is the cochlea. As the surgeon works medially from the otic capsule following the facial nerve, the dissection can be widened to encompass 180° of the IAC. After the IAC has been exposed as widely as possible from the inner ear to the porus acousticus, the dura is opened carefully. The facial nerve is occasionally pressed against the dura by the acoustic neuroma and the nerve can be injured by the dural incision.

After tumor removal is complete and bleeding has been controlled, the IAC is loosely packed with fat, fascia, or muscle. The retractor is removed and the temporal lobe allowed to relax into its normal position. The bone flap is replaced and the temporalis muscle is sutured to the cuff of fascia left along the superior temporal line. (See Table 11–3.)

The approach is hampered by its technical difficulty. Because the surgeon has few guiding landmarks, the structures that the approach is designed to spare, the facial nerve and contents of the otic capsule, can be inadvertently injured. The success in sparing the remaining hearing is mixed, with rates of measurable postoperative hearing ranging from 32–59% (Shelton, Brack-

TABLE 11–3. SUMMARY OF ADVANTAGES AND DISADVANTAGES OF THE MIDDLE CRANIAL FOSSA APPROACH.

Middle Fossa Approach	
Advantages	*Disadvantages*
Hearing preservation	Technically difficult
Largely extradural	Only useful for small tumors
Good exposure of VII	

mann, House, & Hitselberger, 1989b; Gantz, et al., 1986; Glasscock, McKennan, & Levine, 1987; Sanna, et al., 1987).

TRANSLABYRINTHINE APPROACH

Panse in 1904 advocated a translabyrinthine approach which he felt was a more direct approach to the CPA, but which involved the "inevitable destruction of the facial nerve." Of course, this is no longer the case. In many respects, the translabyrinthine approach is the safest approach for removing acoustic neuromas for preservation of the facial nerve. Performed using gouges for bone removal and without the benefit of the surgical microscope, the approach was abandoned prior to 1920. Cushing's (1932) comments about the translabyrinthine approach were "the otologist doubtless will be the first to recognize and diagnose these cases.... But if the otologist has surgical ambitions to treat these lesions there is no possible route more dangerous or difficult than this one."

In 1962, using an operating microscope and an otologic drill, House "rediscovered" the translabyrinthine approach and in 1964 presented what is now recognized as his landmark monograph on the transtemporal approach to the CPA. In his first 54 acoustic neuroma operations, 44 performed via the translabyrinthine approach and 10 performed via the middle cranial fossa approach, there were no deaths. Since these pioneering efforts, the approach has laid to rest the objections raised by Cushing. Although felt by some to be inferior to the suboccipital or retrosigmoid-transmeatal approach in the treatment of large tumors, the translabyrinthine approach allows resection of tumors of any size.

This approach is indicated for tumors of the CPA in patients whose hearing is too poor to warrant a hearing conservation procedure (middle fossa or retrosigmoid-transmeatal). Some surgeons advocate its use in patients with tumors larger than 1.5–2 cm, even in the face of "good" preoperative hearing as few patients with tumors larger than this will have any serviceable hearing when approached through the retrosigmoid-transmeatal or suboccipital procedures (Cohen, Lewis, & Ransohoff, 1993; Kemink, Langman, Niparko, & Graham, 1991). In patients with larger tumors (little chance of hearing preservation), the advantages of the translabyrinthine approach with respect to decreased morbidity and rare mortality outweigh the small chance of hearing preservation offered by other procedures (Tos & Thomsen, 1982).

A C-shaped incision is made in the postauricular skin and the mastoid cortex is exposed (Figure 11–4A). With an otologic drill, a complete mastoidectomy is performed. Bone is removed from the posterior and middle fossa dura. Bone may be left over the sigmoid sinus ("Bill's Island") to prevent it

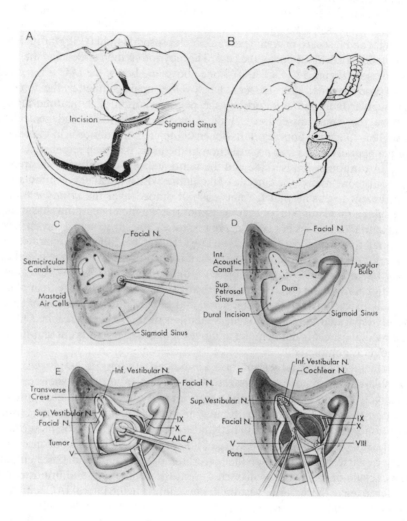

FIGURE 11–4. Translabyrinthine approach to CPA, right ear. **(A)** Site of incision. **(B)** Mastoidectomy. **(C)** Labyrinthectomy. **(D)** Exposure of posterior fossa dura, sigmoid sinus, and internal auditory canal. Note position of mastoid segment of facial nerve. **(E)** Removal of intracapsular tumor contents. **(F)** Removal of final tumor fragments from facial nerve and appearance of operative field after tumor dissection. (From "Microsurgical Anatomy of Acoustic Neuroma" by A. L. Rhoton, Jr., and H. Tedeschi, 1992, *Otolaryngologic Clinics of North America, 25*, p. 291. Copyright 1992 by W. B. Saunders Co. Reprinted by permission.)

from being torn by the spinning shaft of the drill. The incus and the head of malleus are removed and the tendon of the tensor tympani is cut. The "facial recess" is opened, allowing the eustachian tube and middle ear to be packed with fat and fascia to prevent leakage of cerebrospinal fluid (CSF) through the eustachian tube at the end of the case. The labyrinth is then drilled and the IAC is exposed (Figure 11-4, C & D). Bone above and below the IAC is removed to expose the canal 180°. Dissection below the canal is limited by the dome of the jugular bulb and anteriorly by the petrous portion of the carotid artery. Above the canal, dissection is limited by the facial nerve and geniculate ganglion. Once the bone work has been completed, the tumor is in the center of the operative field and no retraction of the brain has been required.

A dural incision is made and the tumor capsule identified at this point. The surgeon "maps" the capsule of the tumor with a facial nerve stimulating instrument to ensure that the nerve is not draped over the *posterior* tumor capsule (a rare situation) or that the tumor is not a facial neuroma. Assuming that stimulation does not elicit nerve responses, the surgeon may, in the case of small tumors, palpate the vertical crest (Bill's bar). Bill's bar separates the superior vestibular from the facial nerve in the lateral IAC. This procedure may be performed with a monopolar stimulating hook to allow functional identification of the facial nerve before any structure is avulsed. A clear plane usually exists between the facial nerve and tumor, allowing the tumor to be gently separated from the facial nerve until its medial aspect is reached. Once the medial aspect is defined, the audiovestibular nerve root is cut and tumor removal is completed.

In the case of larger tumors, a modified strategy is employed. The capsule of the tumor is cauterized with bipolar cautery and incised. The relatively bloodless interior of the tumor may be rapidly and safely "gutted" (Figure 11-4E). A monopolar stimulating instrument helps locate the posterior tumor capsule with the thinned and stretched facial nerve on its surface. As the tumor is gutted, the pressure of the intracranial contents collapses the tumor on itself, allowing even the largest tumor to be removed. Once gutted, the capsule of the tumor is dissected from the cerebellum and brainstem. I prefer to leave the superior vestibular nerve intact in the lateral IAC until this point, as it tends to support the tumor, preventing traction on the facial nerve.

Once the superior vestibular nerve is avulsed from the lateral IAC, the facial nerve can be traced from lateral to medial and tumor capsule resected until the facial nerve becomes indistinguishable from tumor capsule. After the tumor has been debulked, the facial nerve can also be located medially and followed from medial to lateral, resecting the tumor capsule as the structures are separated.

The surgeon treating a large neuroma is often left with the dilemma of a small piece of tumor that cannot be separated from the facial nerve without compromising the integrity of the nerve. Some surgeons, fearing tumor recurrence with incomplete resection, will sacrifice the facial nerve at this point. However, many studies support leaving the remaining facial nerve-tumor capsule intact (*near-total* resection), allowing preservation of facial nerve function (Kemink, LaRouere, Kileny, Telian, & Hoff, 1990; Shea, Hitselberger, Benecke, & Brackmann, 1985). In the vast majority of cases, the tumor capsule is actually devascularized by this time in the surgery and tumor regrowth will not occur. Careful follow-up with serial imaging is mandated in these cases.

The strengths of the translabyrinthine approach are many. The translabyrinthine approach remains extradural until the surgeon is prepared to expose and resect the tumor. The approach limits retraction of the cerebellum and decreases the frequency in which cerebellum must be resected, reducing postoperative morbidity and hospitalization. The translabyrinthine approach places the surgeon at the origin of the tumor and exposes the lateral aspect of the tumor, allowing tumor impacted in the fundus of the IAC to be resected. Most importantly, the approach allows identification of the facial nerve in the IAC where a plane may still be found between the facial nerve and tumor, allowing preservation of the nerve in most cases.

The disadvantages of the translabyrinthine approach are few. The approach necessarily destroys any remaining function of the operated ear. (See Table 11–4.)

STRATEGIES FOR FACIAL NERVE AND HEARING PRESERVATION IN ACOUSTIC NEUROMA SURGERY

The surgical approach to the acoustic tumor is important, as it will likely affect the functional outcome of such neural structures as the facial and

TABLE 11–4. SUMMARY OF ADVANTAGES AND DISADVANTAGES OF THE TRANSLABYRINTHINE APPROACH.

Translabyrinthine Approach	
Advantages	**Disadvantages**
Good exposure	Sacrifices hearing
Early identification of VII	
Largely extradural	
Minimal retraction of cerebellum	

auditory nerves. In the patient with poor preoperative hearing or in patients with serviceable hearing and a tumor with an extracanalicular component protruding farther than 2 cm from the porus acousticus, the translabyrinthine approach is favored.

In patients with tumors that protrude less than 5 mm beyond the porus acousticus and have good preoperative hearing, the middle cranial fossa approach may be chosen, with the understanding that it offers only a 50% chance of any postoperative hearing in well-selected patients. For patients with medium-sized tumors (from 5 mm extension beyond the porus to 2 cm extension) and good preoperative hearing, the retrosigmoid-transmeatal approach may be chosen.

Facial nerve monitoring is useful during acoustic neuroma surgery as an aid to anatomical dissection. Monitoring can identify the location of the nerve before injury is done to the nerve. Through mechanically elicited potentials, monitoring gives the surgeon feedback regarding the effect of surgical maneuvers on the nerve. When using a laser at the end of a case to vaporize and devascularize tumor inseparable from the facial nerve, facial nerve monitoring may indicate heating of the nerve by showing an increasing EMG baseline.

The use of stimulating instruments during dissection further aids the surgeon by allowing exact localization of the nerve when the position of the nerve is distorted by the tumor. Two types of stimulating instruments are currently available. The flush-tip bipolar stimulating instrument performs well, because it limits the spread of stimulating current to surrounding tissues and fluids (Prass & Luders, 1985). Monopolar stimulating instruments, although less accurate in some situations than the bipolar stimulator, allow dissection while the surgeon continuously maps the position of the facial nerve (Kartush, 1989).

Before closing the incision at the end of the procedure, the proximal CN VII is stimulated and the minimum current required to obtain a response is recorded. Beck, Atkins, Benecke, and Brackmann (1991) report that 97% of patients whose facial nerve stimulated at 0.05 mA, yielding a 500 μV contraction on completion of tumor removal, maintained perfect facial results. Some surgeons leave recording electrodes in place as the patient emerges from anesthesia to record voluntary EMG activity that can be helpful in counseling the patient should the patient awake with facial palsy or develop a delayed facial palsy.

Auditory brainstem response (ABR) monitoring is indicated during hearing preservation procedures, although its impact on the surgery remains questionable. Because of the time ABR requires for averaging, ABR does not give real-time feedback of auditory nerve function, unlike facial nerve EMG.

If waves I and V are preserved, there is an excellent chance of hearing preservation and, conversely, if waves I and V are lost there is little chance of hearing preservation (although exceptions have been reported). In practical terms, if during a suboccipital procedure for hearing conservation waves I and V are lost, the surgeon may extend the dissection and perform a "translaby-rinthine drillout" (Poe, Tarlov, & Gadre, 1993) to improve exposure of the lateral IAC and facial nerve.

Some groups routinely perform near-field monitoring of CN VIII function, using electrodes placed on the auditory nerve to give real-time feedback of auditory nerve status. The combination of ABR and near-field recordings may improve outcome, although this, too, is questionable.

The ideal operation for acoustic neuroma removal achieves complete tumor removal while minimizing patient morbidity. These ideals are often met in the resection of small tumors. In large tumors, tissue planes between the tumor and surrounding structures may be obscure. Elderly or medically unstable patients may not tolerate a prolonged anesthetic and speed of resection becomes a greater issue. In these difficult situations, the goal of complete tumor resection may need to be modified. In the symptomatic elderly or medically marginal patient with a large tumor, many surgeons will perform a palliative *subtotal* resection, decompressing the brainstem and cerebellum by removing sufficient tumor while limiting the risk of facial nerve injury (Silverstein, McDaniel, & Wazen, 1985). After subtotal removal, only 15–23% of patients will demonstrate regrowth of tumor and most of these will not require surgery (House, 1968; Wazen et al., 1985). As mentioned earlier, near-total resection (i.e., leaving tumor capsule on the nerve) is reserved for tumors resected to the point where only a rim of capsule densely adherent to the facial nerve remains. A small bit of tumor capsule left on the facial nerve seldom regrows, having been devascularized by the surgery.

CONCLUSIONS

From its origins in 1894, acoustic neuroma surgery has benefited from technologic advances and increased knowledge of anatomy and neurophysiology. The modern collaboration of the surgeon and electrophysiologist allows preservation of neural structures once considered unsalvageable.

REFERENCES

Ballance, C. A. (1907). *Some points in the surgery of the brain and its membranes.* London: MacMillan and Co., Ltd.

Beck, D. L., Atkins, J. S., Benecke, J. E., & Brackmann, D. E. (1991). Intraoperative facial nerve monitoring: Prognostic aspects during acoustic tumor removal. *Otolaryngology—Head and Neck Surgery, 104,* 780–782.

Bell C. (1833). The nervous system of the human body. Washington, D.C.: Green.

Cohen, N. L., Hammerschlag, P. E., Berg, H., & Ransohoff, J. (1986). Acoustic neuroma surgery: An eclectic approach with emphasis on preservation of hearing. The New York University-Bellevue experience. *Annals of Otology, Rhinology, and Laryngology, 95*, 21–29.

Cohen, N. L., Lewis, W. S., & Ransohoff, J. (1993). Hearing preservation in cerebellopontine angle tumor surgery: The NYU experience 1974–1991, *American Journal of Otology, 14*, 423–433.

Cross, J. P. (1981). Unilateral neurilemmomas of the VIIIth cranial nerve: Then and now. *American Journal of Otology, 3*, 28–34.

Cushing, H. (1932). *Intracranial tumors.* Springfield, IL: Charles C. Thomas.

Dandy, W. (1941). Results of removal of acoustic tumors by the unilateral approach. *Archives of Surgery, 42*, 1026–1033.

Dix, M. R., & Hallpike, C. S. (1960). Discussion of acoustic neuroma. *Laryngoscope, 70*, 105–121.

Fraenkel, J., Hunt, J., Woolsey, G., & Elsberg, C. (1904). Contributions to the surgery of neurofibroma of the acoustic nerve with remarks on the surgical procedure. *Annals of Surgery,* 293–319.

Gantz, B. J., Parnes, L. S., Harker, L. A., & McCabe, B. F. (1986). Middle cranial fossa acoustic neuroma excision: Results and complications. *Annals of Otology, Rhinology, and Laryngology, 95*, 454.

Giannotta, S. L., & Pulec, J. L. (1988) Tumors of the cerebellopontine angle: Combined management by neurosurgical and otological surgeons. *Clinical Neurosurgery, 34*, 457–466.

Glasscock, M. E. III, McKennan, K. X., Levine, S. C. (1987). Acoustic neuroma surgery: The results of hearing conservation surgery. *Laryngoscope, 97*, 785.

Henschen, F. (1915). Zur histologie und pathogenes der Kleinhirnbruckenwinkeltumoren. *Archiv Psychiatry, 56*, 21–122.

House, W. F. (1961). Surgical exposure of the internal auditory canal and its contents through the middle cranial fossa. *Laryngoscope, 71*, 1363.

House, W. F. (1962). VIIIth nerve and cochlear surgery in advanced otosclerosis: Preliminary report. In Schuknecht, H. F. (Ed.), *Proceedings of Henry Ford Hospital International Symposium on Otosclerosis* (pp. 371–389). Boston: Little, Brown.

House, W. F. (1964). Report of cases: Transtemporal removal of acoustic neuromas [Monograph]. *Archives of Otolaryngology, 80*, 617.

House, W. (1968). Partial tumor removal and recurrence in acoustic tumor surgery. *Archives of Otolaryngology, 88*, 96–106.

Kartush, J. M. (1989). Electroneuronography and intraoperative facial nerve monitoring in contemporary neurotology. *Otolaryngology—Head and Neck Surgery, 101*, 496–503.

Kartush, J. M., Graham, M. D., LaRouere, M. J. (1991). Meatal decompression following acoustic neuroma resection: Minimizing delayed facial palsy. *Laryngoscope, 101*, 674–675.

Kartush, J. M., Kemink, J. L., Graham, M. D. (1985). The arcuate eminence: Topographic orientation in middle cranial fossa surgery. *Annals of Otology, Rhinology, and Laryngology, 94*, 25–28.

Kemink, J. L., LaRouere, M. J., Kileny, P. R., Telian, S. A., & Hoff, J. T. (1990). Hearing preservation following suboccipital removal of acoustic neuromas. *Laryngoscope, 100*, 597-602.

Kemink, J. L., Langman, A. W., Niparko, J. K., Graham, M. D. (1991). Operative management of acoustic neuromas: The priority of neurologic function over complete resection. *Otolaryngology—Head and Neck Surgery, 104*, 96-99.

Leveque-Lasource, A. (1810). Observation sur un amaurosis et un cophosis, avec perte ou diminution de la voix, des mouvmens, etc, par suite de lesion organique apparente de plusiers parties du serve. *Journale Generale Medicine Chirurgurie Pharmacie, 37*, 368-373.

Panse, R. (1904). Clinical and pathological observations. IV. A glioma of the akusticus. *Archiv Ohrenheilkunde, 61*, 251.

Poe, D. S., Tarlov, E. C., Gadre, A. K. (1993). Translabyrinthine drillout from suboccipital approach to acoustic neuroma. *American Journal of Otology, 14*, 215-219.

Prass, R., & Luders, H. (1985). Constant current versus constant voltage stimulation. *Journal of Neurosurgery, 62*, 622-623.

Rhoton, A. L., Pulec, J., & Hall, G. (1968). Absence of bone over the geniculate ganglion. *Journal of Neurosurgery, 28*, 48-53.

Sanna, M. D., Zini, C., Mazzoni, A., Gandolfi, A., Pareschi R., Pasanisi, E., Gamoletti, R. (1987). Hearing preservation in acoustic neuroma surgery. Middle fossa versus suboccipital approach. *American Journal of Otology, 8*, 500.

Sargent, E. W., Kartush, J. M., & Graham, M. D. (1993). Medial (meatal) facial nerve decompression in acoustic neuroma resection. Unpublished data.

Shea, J. J., Hitselberger, W. E., Benecke, J. E., & Brackmann, D. E. (1985). Recurrence rate of partially resected acoustic tumors. *American Journal of Otology, 107* (Suppl.), 107-109.

Shelton, C., Brackmann, D. E., House, W. F., & Hitselberger W. E. (1989a). Acoustic tumor surgery: Prognostic factors in hearing conservation. *Archives of Otolaryngology—Head and Neck Surgery, 115*, 1213-1216.

Shelton, C., Brackmann, D. E., House, W. F., & Hitselberger W. E. (1989b). Middle fossa acoustic tumor surgery: Results in 106 cases. *Laryngoscope, 99*, 405-408.

Silverstein, H., McDaniel, A., & Wazen, J. (1985). Conservative management of acoustic neuroma in the elderly patient. *Laryngoscope, 95*, 766-770.

Smith, M. F. W., Miller, R. N., & Cox, D. J. (1973). Suboccipital microsurgical removal of acoustic neuromas of all sizes. *Annals of Otology, Rhinology, and Laryngology, 82*, 407-414.

Sterkers, J. M., Perre, J., Viala, P., & Foncin, J.F. (1987). The origin of acoustic neuromas. *Acta Otolaryngologica (Stockholm), 103*, 427-431.

Tos, M., & Thomsen, J. (1982). The price of preservation of hearing in acoustic neuroma surgery. *Annals of Otology, Rhinology, and Laryngology, 91*, 240-245.

Toynbee, J. (1853). Neuroma of the auditory nerve. *Transactions of the Pathology Society of London, 4*, 259-260.

Wazen, J., Silverstein, H., Norrell, H., & Besse, B. (1985). Preoperative and postoperative growth rates in acoustic neuromas documented with CT scanning. *Otolaryngology—Head and Neck Surgery, 93*, 151-155.

■ CHAPTER 12 ■

SPINAL CORD SURGERY

■ RICHARD D. BUCHOLZ, M.D. ■

Spinal surgery consumes the major portion of the time spent in the operating room by most neurosurgeons. As a result of the abnormal stance of homo sapiens on two feet when compared to the rest of the animal world, the human spine is prone to a variety of conditions that require surgical intervention as they are often resistant to medical intervention. Encased within a bony canal, the spinal cord is well protected from external injury, but is uniquely susceptible to degenerative conditions that narrow the diameter of the spinal canal. Neoplastic and infectious processes, although occurring less commonly than degenerative conditions, can also compress the spinal cord, often leading to a rapid and permanent loss of function. The spinal cord itself is extraordinarily sensitive to intraoperative manipulation; it is, therefore, an excellent candidate for intraoperative monitoring. To understand the physiology of spinal monitoring, an understanding of the anatomy, pathology, symptomatology, and surgery of the spinal cord is needed.

SPINAL COLUMN ANATOMY

VERTEBRAL BODY

The spinal column is comprised of 7 cervical, 12 thoracic, and usually 5 lumbar vertebra. Each vertebra, with the exception of the first and second cervical, includes a solid cylindrical anterior section called the vertebral body with a ring-like projection extending posteriorly. The vertebral body is the main structural element of the spine and bears the majority of the weight of the body superior to it. As a reflection of the increased stress on the spine as one descends the spinal column, the vertebral bodies become larger the lower one descends in the spine.

INTERVERTEBRAL DISKS

Between each vertebral body is a cartilaginous structure called the intervertebral disk. The disk serves as a shock absorber for the rest of the spine. Within each disk is a somewhat gelatinous substance called the nucleus pulposus, which is confined to the center of the disk by the ligamentous annulus fibrosus. Should the axial stress on the disk exceed the ability of the annulus to confine the nucleus pulposus, this material will rupture through the annulus, forming a herniated or ruptured disk (Figure 12-1).

PEDICLES

The ring-like projection from the posterior aspect of the vertebral body is made up of several elements (Figure 12-2). The ring protects the spinal cord and also provides two additional joints (the facets), which connect the vertebra to the rest of the spinal column. The ring is connected to the vertebral body by two pedicles, which are round in cross section, that attach the facets to the vertebral body.

FACET JOINTS

Each vertebra has four facet joints, with a pair on each side of the ring. Each pair of facets has two articular surfaces, with one surface directed superiorly to touch the vertebra above and the other exposed inferiorly, to relate to the vertebra below. The facet joints carry the remainder of the weight not born by the vertebral bodies and like the vertebral bodies increase in size as one descends from the top of the spinal column to the lumbar area. Each pair of facet joints is connected by a strong bony strut, the pars interarticularis, that can be congenitally absent, leading to a slippage of the bodies termed spondylolisthesis (Figure 12-3).

TRANSVERSE PROCESSES

Projecting out laterally from the facet joints are bony struts called the transverse processes (Figure 12-2). These processes serve as attachment sites

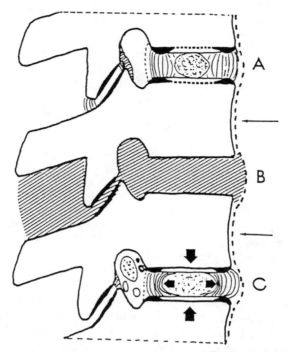

FIGURE 12–1. Sagittal view of the medial aspect of the spinal column, showing the intervertebral disk and herniated nucleus pulposus. (From *The Spine* by S. Rothman and S. Simeone. Philadelphia: W. B. Saunders Company, 2nd edition, 1982. Reprinted by permission.)

for the extensive paravertebral muscles and in the thoracic level articulate with the ribs. Surgeons use these processes to attach bone grafts and instrumentation to fuse the spine.

LAMINA

Completing the posterior half of the ring is a thin, shell-like bone called the lamina (Figure 12–2). The lamina of neighboring vertebra overlap, protecting the spinal cord from penetrating injury. From the midsection of each lamina a projection arises, called the spinous process, which serves as an attachment site for paravertebral muscles in a manner similar to the transverse processes. The spinous process divides the lamina into two equal halves, the hemilam-

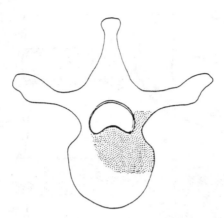

FIGURE 12-2. Superior view of a typical vertebral body, demonstrating the (1) pedicles, (2) transverse processes, and (3) lamina. (From *The Spine* by S. Rothman and S. Simeone. Philadelphia: W. B. Saunders Company, 2nd edition, 1982. Reprinted by permission.)

ina. To expose the posterior aspect of the spinal cord to remove a laterally situated lesion such as a herniated disk, either a portion (hemilaminotomy) or the entirety of one hemilamina (hemilaminectomy) is removed. If the spinal cord or nerve roots are compressed from a central process, or the pathology lies within the coverings of the spinal cord, the entire lamina and spinous process is removed in a procedure called a laminectomy.

SPINAL CORD ANATOMY

MENINGES

The spinal cord is enveloped by three layers of coverings, which provide a barrier to disease and contain the cerebrospinal fluid that suspends the neural elements. The toughest of these layers, the dura, effectively segregates disease into extradural and intradural processes, as few disease entities can penetrate this tough membrane. Intradural processes can be further divided into extramedullary processes, which are outside the spinal cord, and intramedullary processes, lesions which arise from or in the parenchyma of the spinal cord.

Spinal Cord

The spinal cord is oval in cross section and has a varying diameter as it progresses from the top of the spinal canal to its termination at the second lumbar vertebra. The cord is tethered laterally to the dura by tissue append-

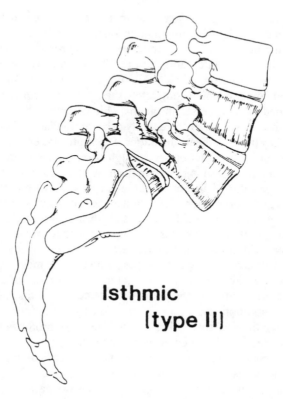

Isthmic (type II)

FIGURE 12–3. Lateral view of lumbar spine with congenital absence of the pars interarticularis resulting in spondylolisthesis (From *The Spine* by S. Rothman and S. Simeone. Philadelphia: W. B. Saunders Company, 2nd edition, 1982. Reprinted by permission.)

ages called the dentate ligaments. For its entire length, the spinal cord gives off nerve roots at four points along its circumference, two anterior and two posterior. These nerve roots come off in pairs, left and right, with the anterior roots serving primarily a motor function, with impulses leaving the spinal cord to actuate muscles. The posterior nerve roots are primarily sensory in nature and bring sensory information from various receptors to the central nervous system (CNS). The posterior roots have a swelling in them about 1.5 cm beyond their exit point from the spinal cord, called the dorsal root ganglion, which is the repository of the cell bodies of neurons conveying sensory information. This structure is removed surgically in an attempt to relieve pain in an area of skin innervated by the nerve root called a dermatome.

The spinal cord consists of two distinct elements, the centrally located gray matter encircled by the white matter. As in the brain, the gray matter is made of a dense network of cell connections and neuronal cell bodies, called the neuropil, where the integration of the CNS occurs. The gray matter is responsible for all the communications within a specific segment of the spinal cord. The white matter, which completely surrounds the neuropil, consists of long cellular neuronal processes, the axons, which represent the long-distance pathways of the CNS. There is essentially no communication between these pathways as they travel in the white matter. The white matter is more resistant to injury than the grey matter either through compression or deprivation of blood flow. Therefore, cord injuries can occur with a local loss of function at the level damaged, due to disruption of the gray matter, with preservation of the long tracts and preservation of function in the lower spinal cord segments. This pattern of injury is called the central cord syndrome, as it reflects selective damage to the center of the cord and the gray matter.

The fibers within the white matter are arranged in specific pathways called tracts. Although there are numerous pathways, the most important are the spinothalamic tract, situated in the anterior portion of the cord, which transmits pain information to the brain; the fasciculus gracilis and cuneatus, which convey vibration and position sensation from the leg and the arm, respectively; and the corticospinal pathways, the major motor systems of the body through which the brain controls movement.

This grouping of pathways into tracts is of critical importance in determining the symptoms and signs of a particular spinal cord injury. It is of great importance to note that the monitoring of sensory pathways, which are generally located anteriorly in the cord, with somatosensory evoked potentials (SSEPs) will not comment on what might be occurring to the posterior aspect of the spinal cord, where the critical motor pathways are located. Relying on SSEP data alone for monitoring may therefore result in a patient who emerges from surgery with a devastating paralysis.

PATHOLOGY

Anatomy provides a mechanism for the organization of the pathology of the spine. As with all organs, the spine can be damaged by trauma, loss of blood flow, infection, or degeneration. As the anatomy of the pathological process will dictate which spinal structures are injured and, therefore, the signs of the disease and response to surgery, it is useful to group pathological processes by location, rather than by etiology. As mentioned previously, the dura provides a barrier to disease and can also serve in categorizing spinal pathology.

EXTRADURAL

Common extradural conditions include degeneration or arthritis of the surrounding spinal column or joints. Such degeneration usually consists of bony protrusions from the joints called bone spurs. This condition, when generalized over several levels, is termed spondylosis. The spinal cord is particularly susceptible to degenerative compression if the spinal canal is congenitally small, called spinal stenosis, a condition that can affect the entire canal or be limited to specific spinal segments. Compression can also occur by an infection within the disk space or vertebral body usually caused by either staphylococcal septicemia or tuberculosis respectively. Metastatic neoplasia typically destroys the vertebral body, resulting in a compression fracture with compression of the neural elements by bone fragments. Herniated disks can mimic neoplasms by compressing single nerve roots or, if more centrally located, compressing the canal itself. One of the most common mechanisms for extradural compression of the spinal cord is seen following injury, with compression or disruption of the cord caused by bony elements driven into the canal, slippage of the vertebral bodies, or by hemorrhage into the canal.

INTRADURAL EXTRAMEDULLARY

Diseases within the dura usually arise either from the coverings of the cord or the intradural portion of the nerve roots. Tumors arising from the nerve roots, as they cross the intradural extramedullary space, are the most frequently seen pathological process in this location. The two common types of tumors in this location are benign neurofibromas or meningiomas. Neurofibromas arising from the nerve roots can be solitary or multiple, a condition usually seen with neurofibromatosis (von Recklinghausen's disease) in which neurofibromas are disseminated throughout the body. Meningiomas are benign tumors that arise from the coverings of the spinal cord and compress the cord from any quadrant.

INTRAMEDULLARY

Intramedullary processes are usually a result of neoplasia or degeneration of the spinal cord itself. Examples of intrinsic neoplasia of spinal cord include gliomas, tumors of the supportive elements of the nervous system, which are usually benign and amenable to complete resection, or ependymomas, which can either arise in the spine or spread to there from a site elsewhere in the CNS, which carry a poor prognosis. The most common degenerative condition of the spinal cord is syringomyelia, in which the gray matter deteriorates and is replaced by a large cyst, which can lead to white matter dysfunction by compression from within. The cause of this degeneration is unknown, but the condition seems to respond to drainage of the cyst fluid into either the subarachnoid or intraperitoneal space (Figure 12–4).

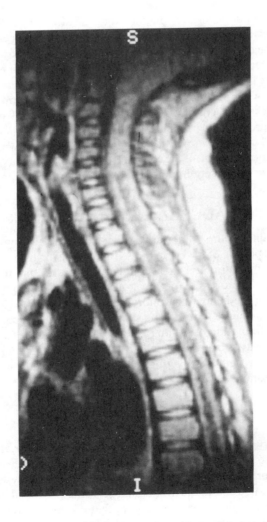

FIGURE 12–4. Sagittal magnetic resonance image of syringomyelia of the cervical spinal cord enlarged by a large syrinx. (From *Review of Medical Physiology* by W. F. Ganong. Norwalk, CT: Appleton & Lange, 1993. Reprinted by permission.)

CLINICAL PRESENTATION

An abnormality within the spinal column comes to the attention of the patient because of compression of the spinal cord or its roots or by an irritation of the pain fibers innervating the vertebra. The diagnosis of spinal column pathology can be based either on subjective complaints expressed by the patient, termed symptoms, or by objective findings (called signs) demonstrated by a physician at the time of examination. It is very important to distinguish between symptoms and signs, as the vast majority of patients have many symptoms that suggest spinal pathology, but few manifest the objective signs of spinal dysfunction. The outcome from surgery is generally greatly enhanced by the presence of preoperative objective findings.

SYMPTOMS

By far the most common presenting symptom of back problems is pain. It has been estimated that up to 75% of all individuals experience back pain at some time during their life. Spinal pain can be classified as either local, located directly over the vertebra themselves, or radicular, extending over the distribution of a spinal nerve root. The most common radicular pain is located over the posterior aspect of the leg and is called sciatica after the nerve that innervates this area. Radicular pain is usually more intense and closer to the spine and rarely involves the most distal aspect of the extremities. Another common symptom seen frequently with pain is spasm in the paravertebral musculature, or "catching" of their back, suggestive of spinal instability. Other symptoms suggest spinal nerve root dysfunction, such as numbness, weakness, tingling, or burning. The value of such symptoms in indicating disease that may be amenable to surgical intervention is greatly enhanced if the symptoms seem to follow a specific dermatome or nerve. Finally, any history of bladder or bowel dysfunction, especially incontinence, is important to elicit, which suggests severe spinal cord compression.

SIGNS

Objective findings indicating spinal cord function can be grouped to reflect if the sign is caused by malfunction of the white or gray matter or by compression of the nerve roots. Gray matter or nerve root involvement will usually cause abnormalities in one of two spinal levels and is termed radiculopathy. White matter dysfunction will be manifested by abnormalities of function at a site distant to the level of involvement and is termed myelopathy. In general, radicular processes respond to surgical intervention more readily than do myelopathic ones.

RADICULOPATHY

By definition radiculopathic abnormalities are confined to a specific spinal segment. The sensory segments are fairly well defined in humans. Sensory signs are elicited by touching the patient with a sharp object to test pain, a vibrating object (such as a tuning fork) to test vibration, and by asking the patient to detect small changes in the angle of the joints with the eyes closed to test proprioception, or by checking the person's sensation of position. Although such sensory findings are deemed "objectives," they rely upon the patient to convey what they are feeling, which can be quite subjective. Motor abnormalities, on the other hand, are more objective, with an examiner rating the strength of each individual muscle tested on a 5-point scale (Table 12-1). The muscles can be grouped by their respective root innervation and an examiner should attempt to decide which root or roots are involved by assaying the strength of all major muscle groups (Table 12-2). As part of the motor examination, the monosynaptic reflexes should be obtained by tapping the muscle tendons with a reflex hammer. These reflexes are orchestrated by sensory input coming from the muscle to the spinal cord, which synapses within the anterior horn of the cord upon motor neurons that control the muscle tested (Figure 12-5). The reflexes orchestrated at or immediately below the level of a pathological process will either be diminished or absent. Far below the level of involvement, if there is damage to the corticospinal pathways that inhibit this monosynaptic reflex, there can be exaggerated reflexes (hyperreflexia), which is a sign of myelopathy.

MYELOPATHY

Other myelopathic signs, like hyperreflexia, can be differentiated from radiculopathy in that entire extremities are involved, as opposed to specific spinal segments as in radiculopathy. For example, damage to the spinothalamic tracts in the cervical region will result in a loss of pinprick in both lower extremities. Occasionally, with extensive damage to spinal pathways that control the motor systems through inhibitory output from the CNS, spontaneous involuntary movements can occur called spasticity, which can be quite distressing to an individual. Such involuntary movements affect not only the skeletal muscle, but can affect the bladder, causing incontinence (an involuntary emptying of the bladder or bowel) and abnormal reflexes, such as the Babinski sign, all indicating loss of cortical control.

CLINICAL GROUPINGS OF SIGNS AND SYMPTOMS

In general, the anatomy of a pathological process can be ascertained by associating the patient's symptoms with the signs found on examination.

TABLE 12–1. GRADING OF MUSCLE STRENGTH.

Grade 0	0% Zero (O)	No evidence of contractility.
Grade 1	10% Trace (T)	Slight contractility, but no joint motion.
Grade 2	25% Poor (P)	Complete motion with gravity eliminated.
Grade 3	50% Fair (F)	Rarely complete motion against gravity.
Grade 4	75% Good (G)	Complete motion against gravity and some resistance.
Grade 5	100% Normal (N)	Complete motion against gravity and full resistance.

Lateral, extradural processes classically compress one or more nerve roots ipsilaterally and result in radiculopathy. As the nerve roots are more resistant to injury than the cord, one can expect good recovery of function lost prior to surgery. More centrally located processes, especially trauma, usually inflict damage on the white matter pathways, with resultant myelopathy. These myelopathic signs may be accompanied by localized trauma to the local nerve roots with an isolated radiculopathy, as well. Diseases arising within the cord, such as the degeneration of the gray matter seen in syringomyelia, result in segmented malfunction and appear in early stages as a radiculopathy. This situation is differentiated from the extradural process discussed above by the fact that the radiculopathy is bilateral. These conditions are not associated with the optimistic prognosis reserved for more laterally situated pathology.

The response to surgery is dictated by many factors, such as age, pre-existing medical conditions, nutrition, and delay in diagnosis. Although the anatomy of the pathological process is important in determining the response to surgery, time is even great importance. The longer a process is allowed to proceed and the more extensive the neurological deficit, the less likely and extensive the recovery.

SURGERY

GOALS

Spinal surgery is advised usually for one of two reasons. The goal of surgery is either to decompress the spinal cord by opening the spinal canal, and possibly removing what is causing compression and neurological symptoms, or to stabilize the spine, repairing instability produced either by degeneration, infection, neoplasia, or surgery. This duality of purpose can be used to classify spinal surgery. Generally, decompressive surgery is performed by the removal of tissue, whereas corrective, stabilizing surgery is performed by the addition of stabilizing material—either bone, plastic, or metal.

TABLE 12–2. MAJOR MUSCLES AND ROOT INNERVATION.

Arm, elevation and rotation:	Deltoideus (axillary nerve from C-5 to C-6)
Elbow, flexion:	Biceps brachii, Brachialis (musculocutaneous nerve from C-5 to C-6)
Elbow, extension:	Triceps brachii (radial nerve from C-7 to T-1)
Elbow, pronation:	Pronator teres (median nerve from C-6 to C-7)
Wrist, extension and abduction:	Extensor carpi ulnaris (radial nerve from C-7 to C-8)
Thumb, extension of distal phalanx:	Extensor pollicis longus (radial nerve from C-7 to C-8)
Thumb, flexion of proximal phalanx:	Flexor pollicis longus et brevis (median nerve from C-7 to T-1)
Fingers, adduction of four fingers:	Interossei palmares (ulnar nerve from C-8 to T-1)
Fingers, abduction of four fingers:	Interossei dorsales (ulnar nerve from C-8 to T-1)
Hip, flexion:	Iliacus (femoral nerve), Psoas (L-2 to L-3), Sartorius (femoral nerve from L-2 to L-3)
Hip, extension:	Gluteus maximus (inferior gluteal nerve from L-4 or S-2), Adductor magnus (sciatic nerve and obturator nerve from L-5 to S-2)
Hip, abduction:	Gluteus medius (superior gluteal nerve from L-4 to S-1), Gluteus maximus (inferior gluteal nerve from L-4 to S-2)
Hip, adduction:	Adductor magnus (sciatic and obturator nerves from L-5 to S-2)
Knee, flexion:	Biceps femoris, Semitendinosus, Semimembranosus, Gastrocnemius (all through sciatic nerve from L-5 to S-2)
Knee, extension:	Quadriceps femoris (femoral nerve from L-2 to L-4)
Ankle, plantar flexion:	Tibialis posterior (posterior tibial nerve from L-5 to S-3), Peroneus longus et brevis (superficial peroneal nerve from L-5 to S-2), Flexor digitorum longus (posterior tibial nerve from S-1 to S-2)
Ankle, dorsiflexion:	Tibialis anterior (deep peroneal nerve from L-4 to S-2)
Foot, inversion:	Tibialis anterior (deep peroneal nerve from L-4 to S-2)
Foot, eversion:	Peroneus longus (superficial peroneal nerve from L-5 to S-2)

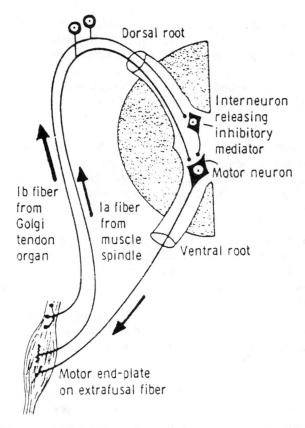

FIGURE 12–5. Diagram of a typical monosynaptic reflex arc, with a sensory neuron, a synapse, and a motor neuron. (From *Review of Medical Physiology* by W. F. Ganong. Norwalk, CT: Appleton & Lange, 1993. Reprinted by permission.)

CLASSIFICATION

Surgery can be further classified by the route of the planned procedure. Throughout its length, the spine can be approached in two ways, anteriorly or posteriorly. The anterior route requires removal of at least an intervertebral disk and occasionally a vertebral body, to expose the anterior surface of the spinal cord. In the posterior approach, the spine is visualized following a partial or total removal of the posterior elements, called the lamina. The choice between these approaches is usually dictated by the anatomy of the pathology, as anterior lesions cannot be approached posteriorly. The exception to this rule is in the lowermost recesses of the spine where the cord has already terminated and the cauda equina can be retracted safely to expose anteriorly based pathology. If the lesion can be safely removed by either approach, posterior surgery is preferred, as it involves less dissection and generally affords a better exposure up and down the spine.

Anterior

Surgery performed through an anterior route is usually in response to a herniated disk in the cervical or thoracic spine, an anteriorly situated bone spur, or a process affecting the vertebral body, such as neoplasia or infection. The technique of anterior approach varies with the portion of the column involved.

STRAIGHT ANTERIOR.   The cervical spine can be exposed through a direct anterior dissection between the esophagus and trachea in the midline and the carotid and strap muscles, laterally. The disk or vertebral body is then removed piecemeal, starting from the front and moving posteriorly toward the spinal canal. Anterior surgery is somewhat more complex, as a large amount of bone or tissue has to be removed prior to visualization of the spinal canal. Care must be taken in removing this tissue, as breaking through the most posterior aspect of the vertebral body can cause the surgeon to fall into the canal with potentially disastrous result.

MODIFIED LATERAL: TRANS THORACIC VERTEBRECTOMY.   In the thoracic spine, the presence of the heart and the great vessels precludes a direct anterior approach. Instead, the surgeon can take advantage of the thoracic cavity to expose the spine from the anterio-lateral aspect. One lung is deflated using a specially designed endotracheal tube that separately aerates the lungs. An incision is made in the anterior portion of the lateral chest wall and a rib is removed to gain access to the thoracic cavity. Surgery is performed through the thorax on the anterior margin of the vertebral column, in a fashion analogous to the cervical procedure. The major drawback to this procedure is that the surgeon is working at some distance from the spinal column, making the surgery technically difficult. To adequately decompress the anterior canal, a disk and usually an invertebral body has to be removed, and replacement with some sort of strut graph is usually required.

POSTEROLATERAL APPROACH: COSTOTRANSVERSECTOMY.   The posterolateral approach can address the problems of the lateral approach. An incision is made off midline on the posterior chest wall and the spine visualized by removing the proximal rib and the transverse process. By dissecting through the paravertebral musculature, the head of the rib can be seen and the vertebral body removed, starting at the point from which the transverse process emanates. The benefit of this procedure, besides that the surgeon does not have to work at depth, is that the spinal canal is seen early and can be used as a landmark to avoid inadvertent penetration into the canal. The drawback of the procedure is that the anterior aspect of the canal is seen at best only tangentially and that compression arising from the opposite side of the vertebral body can be difficult to remove.

STABILIZATION TECHNIQUES. After any anterior approach, the spine is left in a precarious situation. Usually the anterior and posterior longitudinal ligaments, as well as a disk or vertebral body, have been removed, leaving a large void. The traditional approach to this problem has been to replace the removed tissue using a strut of bone taken from the patient's hip. The bone is usually wedged into the void while distracting the spine and held in place by removing the distraction and using the weight of the body to maintain position. As a response to the complication of extrusion of these struts, new instrumentation has been devised that stabilizes the strut with screws and stainless steel bars.

Posterior

The posterior approach is greatly preferred to decompress or expose vast expanses of the spine. The degree of decompression is tailored to the extensiveness of the disease involved.

HEMILAMINECTOMY. The most common posterior procedure is to remove herniated disks. As these lesions are usually laterally situated, a portion of the lamina is removed (hemilaminectomy). This limited approach affords good visualization of a single nerve root, and by retracting the nerve root medially, the anterior aspect of the spinal canal can be inspected to ensure that no additional fragments are present. By limiting the procedure, postoperative pain is reduced, instability is minimized, and fusion is rarely needed. If multiple levels are involved, multiple hemilaminectomies can be performed, but it is decidedly unusual for multiple disk herniations to occur simultaneously at different levels.

LAMINECTOMY. For conditions that involve both sides of the spinal canal, or when the canal has been narrowed, adequate decompression can be obtained only by removing the entire lamina in a laminectomy. For the majority of cases, simple removal of the lamina or multiple laminae is sufficient to decompress the spinal canal, as is the case with spinal stenosis. Multiple level laminectomies are also performed when the pathology is located intradurally, as it is the only procedure that affords adequate exposure to enter the spinal cord. During such a procedure the dura is opened parallel to the long axis of the spinal cord and, if the pathology is located within the cord, the posterior sulcus of the spinal cord is dissected to obtain intraspinal access. Instability is usually not seen after a simple laminectomy, unless the surgery is performed in the cervical spine of an infant or if the decompression requires the removal of one or more facet joints.

FUSION.   Fusion is usually only necessary with trauma, extensive degeneration of the spine, or in metastatic neoplasia. A variety of fusion techniques have been developed and new instrumentation is appearing almost daily. In the past, long cylindrical rods equipped with hooks that wrap around the lamina were used to stabilize the spine. Although still used for fusions over multiple levels, rods are now employed less commonly because their high failure rate and a tendency to accelerate degeneration of the spine above and below the level of the fusion. Smaller plates attached to the spine using screws placed through the pedicle of the vertebra are currently used. These short fusions are usually combined with the placement of bone on the adjacent transverse processes to further stabilize the spine. The major complications of such a fusion are the risk of impaling a nerve root by poor placement of a screw or mechanical failure of the plate.

MONITORING

Inasmuch as the primary function of the spinal cord is to convey sensory and motor information, there are two categories of function that can be monitored during spinal surgery. Sensory function is more commonly monitored, as it is relatively simple to evoke and record sensory impulses in the cord during anesthesia. However, as far as the patient is concerned, a motor deficit is far more important than any sensory loss. Therefore, there is a continuing search for techniques to produce and record motor impulses within the CNS.

Sensory

The most common technique to monitor sensory functions is through the use of somatosensory evoked potentials (SSEPs). A nerve distal to the level of surgery is stimulated by a small current induced between two electrodes. The ascent of the resultant evoked potential can be recorded directly from the cortex, using electrodes positioned over the central sulcus or by electrodes located over the spinal cord. As these potentials are small, and the noise level in the operating room fairly large, many potentials have to be added together to cancel out background noise. A major disadvantage of evoked potential monitoring is the delay imposed in detecting a change by using an averaging process. Another disadvantage is that extensive damage can occur to the posteriorly located motor pathways without any change in the SSEP which is transmitted in the anterior portion of the cord.

Motor

Recent work has focused on the possibility of stimulating the motor pathways. One technique involves the use of a strong pulsing magnetic field that can evoke activity in the motor cortex without penetrating the skull with an electrode. These magnetic fields, generated by small ring magnets, can produce a motor contraction that can be recorded distal to the site of surgery. The major drawbacks of this form of monitoring are the problems associated with using these strong temporary magnetic fields in the operating room and maintaining the magnet in a fixed position directly over the motor cortex. In addition, the motor potentials produced are small and require averaging as with SSEPs, with the attendant delay in diagnosis should function fail.

CONCLUSIONS

The spine is a frequent target of neurosurgeons and orthopedists. It is prone to injury and tolerates compression poorly. Its extreme sensitivity to manipulation and the disastrous results of such manipulation make it imperative that the function of the cord is continuously monitored intraoperatively. The use of functional spinal monitoring will be enhanced by improvements and much wider use in the near future.

ACKNOWLEDGMENT

The MR of syringomyelia was kindly provided by Dr. David Martin, Department of Radiology, St. Louis University Health Sciences Center, St. Louis, Missouri.

REFERENCES

Degowan, X., & Degowan, X. (1969). *Bedside diagnostic examination.* New York: Macmillan.
Ganon, W. F. (1993). *Review of medical physiology.* Norwalk, CT: Appleton & Lange.
Rothman, S., & Simeone, S. (1982). *The spine* (2nd Ed.). Philadelphia: W. B. Saunders.

CHAPTER 13

ANESTHESIA AND INTRAOPERATIVE MONITORING

■ SANDRA B. KINSELLA, M.D. ■

Anesthesia is defined as the insensibility, general or local, induced by anesthetic agents, hypnosis, or acupuncture as well as the loss of sensation of neurogenic or psychogenic origin. The anesthesiologist has the responsibility to render the patient insensible of pain during surgical, obstetrical, therapeutic, and diagnostic procedures. Therefore, there is an interrelationship between the giving of anesthetic drugs and the ability to perform intraoperative nerve monitoring.

This chapter describes this relationship. Sensory evoked potentials (SEP) and motor evoked potentials (MEP) will be addressed. There is a large armamentarium of anesthetic drugs available in 1994 that has an effect on intraoperative nerve monitoring. Multiple anesthetic techniques are available. The choice of technique depends on many variables, including patient condition, surgical procedure, and anesthesiologist preference. The three most common techniques are the inhalation technique, the balanced technique, and the high-dose narcotic technique.

The inhalation technique uses one of the volatile anesthetics (halothane, enflurane, or isoflurane), frequently in conjunction with nitrous oxide. Low doses of narcotics may be given as boluses to supplement the anesthetic depth.

The balanced technique consists mainly of narcotics, such as morphine sulfate, fentanyl, sufentanil, alfentanyl, and the non-narcotic agent, propofol, administered by a continuous infusion or by repetitive bolusing, combined with nitrous oxide. A volatile agent could also be used to supplement as needed.

Finally, the high-dose narcotic technique, which is often used in patients with heart disease, uses very large dosages of narcotics given by continuous infusion or by repetitive bolus. Nitrous oxide and/or volatile agents can also be used with this technique. With any of the three anesthetic techniques there will be alterations made, depending on the needs of the patient as they change throughout the surgical procedure.

MAC is a term used by anesthesiologists when discussing volatile anesthetics. MAC is minimum alveolar concentration (partial pressure) of an inhaled anesthetic at 1 atmosphere expressed in percentage of concentration that prevents skeletal muscle movement in response to a noxious stimulus (surgical incision) in 50% of patients (Stoelting & Miller, 1984). Throughout this chapter, the volatile anesthetics, and nitrous oxide, will be described as MAC or in percentage.

SENSORY EVOKED POTENTIALS

There are three commonly monitored sensory evoked potentials. These are the somatosensory evoked potentials (SSEP), visual evoked potentials (VEP), and the auditory brainstem responses (ABR). The details of the monitoring of these evoked potentials are described in other chapters of this book.

Briefly, the sensory stimulus is generated and the audiologist watches for changes from baseline in the latency, amplitude, or morphology of the waveform. Any changes from baseline may indicate to the surgeon the possibility of having violated the integrity of the nerve or nerve pathway.

All SEPs are affected by the anesthetic agents (see Table 13–1). The VEPs are the most sensitive and the ABRs are the least sensitive to anesthetic drugs. Also, the early potentials are less sensitive to anesthetics than are the late potentials (Black & Cucchiara, 1990; Peterson, Drummond, & Todd, 1986).

It is noteworthy that the selection of drugs and the dosing of drugs may change during the course of the surgery. This will occur as the level of surgical stimulation changes along with changes in the patient's vital signs. The audiologist is advised to communicate throughout the case with the anesthesiologist.

Volatile anesthetics can be used when monitoring SSEP, but they have been shown to cause a dose-dependant increase in latency and a decrease in amplitude as shown in Figure 13–1 (Bendo, Kass, Hartung, & Cottrell, 1992;

TABLE 13–1. ANESTHETIC DRUG EFFECTS ON SEPs.

Drugs	ABR Latency	ABR Amplitude	SSEPs Latency	SSEPs Amplitude	VEP Latency	VEP Amplitude
Thiopental						
4-6 mg/kg	0	0	0	0	—	—
20 mg/kg	↑	0	↑	↓	↑	↓
75 mg/kg	↑	↓	↑	↓	↑	↓
Pentobarbital						
9-18 mg/kg	↑	↓	↑	↑	↑	↓
Droperidol						
0.1 mg/kg	—	—	↑	↓	—	—
Diazepam						
0.1 mg/kg	0	0	↑	↓	—	—
Midazolam	—	—	0	↓	—	—
Meperidine	—	—	↑	↑/↓	—	—
Morphine	—	—	↑	↓	—	—
Fentanyl	0	0	↑	↓	—	—
Sufentanil	0	0	0	↓	—	—
Alfentanil	0	0	0	↓	—	—
Etomidate						
0.05-0.3 mg/kg/min	0	0	↑	↑	—	—
Propofol						
2-6 mg/kg	0	0	↑	↓	—	—
Enflurane	↑	0	↑	↓*	↑	↓
Halothane	↑	0	↑	↓	↑	0

continued

TABLE 13–1. *(continued)*

Drugs	ABR Latency	ABR Amplitude	SSEPs Latency	SSEPs Amplitude	VEP Latency	VEP Amplitude
Isoflurane	↑	0	↑	↓*	↑	↓
Nitrous Oxide	0	0	0	↓	↑	↓

ABR = Auditory Brainstem Responses, SSEP = Somatosensory Evoked Potentials, VEP = Visual Evoked Potentials, ↑ = increase, ↓ = decrease, 0 = no change, — = no data.
* 1.5 MAC enflurane and isoflurane (but not halothane) will occasionally abolish the cortical evoked response to median nerve stimulation. *Source:* Adapted from "Neurophysiology and Neuroanesthesia" by A. Bendo, I. Kass, J. Hartung, and J. Cottrell (p. 884) in *Clinical Anesthesia,* P. Barash, B. Cullen, and R. Stoelting (Eds.), 1992, Philadelphia: J. B. Lippincott Company. Copyright 1992 by J. B. Lippincott Company. Adapted by permission. Also: adapted from "Neurologic Monitoring" by S. Black and R. Cucchiara (p. 1334) in *Anesthesia,* R. Miller (Ed.), 1994, New York: Churchill Livingstone. Copyright 1994 by Churchill Livingstone Inc. Adapted by permission.

Black & Cucchiara, 1990). The literature is not consistent as to which volatile anesthetic has the greater effect on the SSEP. Some studies show that halothane has a greater effect than enflurane or isoflurane on SSEP, but other studies show the opposite.

Acceptable conditions for monitoring cortical SSEP exist with isoflurane at 0.5–1 MAC with nitrous oxide; and are probably the same for enflurane and halothane (Black & Cucchiara, 1990). Higher concentrations of all volatile anesthetics will eliminate cortical sensory evoked potentials (Bendo et al., 1992).

Nitrous oxide, a nonvolatile anesthetic, which is used in many anesthetics in conjunction with another anesthetic agent, also has an effect on SSEP. Nitrous oxide causes a decrease in amplitude without a change in latency when added to either a narcotic or inhalational anesthetic (Black & Cucchiara, 1990). This effect is often more pronounced in patients with abnormal preoperative SSEP (Black & Cucchiara, 1990). Nitrous oxide, when used alone, caused an increase in latency and decrease in amplitude when monitoring VEP (Black & Cucchiara, 1990).

The inhalation anesthetics have less of an effect on the ABR. When these agents are used in routine concentrations, there is an increase in latency with little to no change in amplitude (Black & Cucchiara, 1990). There will be an

Anesthesiology
V 65, No 1, Jul 1986

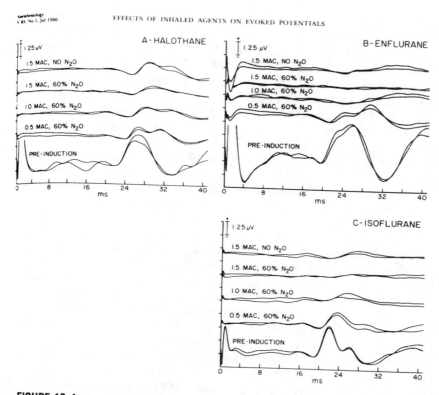

FIGURE 13-1. Representative SSEP cortical responses C-3' or C-4' — FPz) at various MAC levels of halothane (A), enflurane (B), and isoflurane (C) with 60% N_2O, and at 1.5 MAC without N_2O.

increase in latency and a decrease in amplitude in the early cortical responses (Black & Cucchiara, 1990).

The effects of the volatile anesthetics on the VEP include a dose-dependent increase in latency, with or without changes in the amplitude of the response (Black & Cucchiara, 1990). Isoflurane at an end-tidal concentration of 1.2% will completely abolish the VEP (McPherson, 1993).

The intravenous anesthetic agents are numerous and may be given at variable times during the procedure. As can be recognized from Table 13-1, many drugs have been evaluated in conjunction with intraoperative monitoring. Some agents, thiopental, etomidate and propofol, are predominantly used for the induction of anesthesia. Other intravenous agents are used to maintain the anesthetic, either by repeat bolus injection or by continuous infusion. Included in this latter group are fentanyl, sufentanil, alfentanil, and propofol.

The usual induction dose of thiopental will not affect SSEP (Bendo et al., 1992); however, larger amounts of thiopental cause a dose-dependent increase in latency and decrease in amplitude in SSEP and an increase in latency of the ABR (Bendo et al., 1992; Black & Cucchiara, 1990). VEPs are the most sensitive of the SEPs to thiopental and at low doses of thiopental, all but the earliest of potentials are lost (Bendo et al., 1992; Black & Cucchiara, 1990). SSEPs are maintained with induction doses of etomidate (Bendo et al., 1992). With either bolus dosing or infusions of etomidate, there is an increase in latency and an increase in amplitude of cortical SSEP with a slight decrease in cervical potentials (Bendo et al., 1992; Black & Cucchiara, 1990). The effect of etomidate on the ABR is similar to the inhalational agents, with an increase in latency and a decrease in amplitude in the early cortical peaks, but without any effect on the brainstem peaks (Navartnarajah, Thorton, Heneghan, Bateman, & Jones, 1983).

Narcotic agents are given by repetitive bolus or continuous infusion and may be used as the main anesthetic or to augment an inhalation anesthetic. Morphine and fentanyl cause an increase in latency and decrease in amplitude (Bendo et al., 1992; Black & Cucchiara, 1990; Grundy, 1980; Pathak, Brown, Cascorbi, & Nash, 1984), although the changes in amplitude are less consistent. Fentanyl has a greater effect on the cortical waves. In a study of nine patients undergoing cardiac surgery, all of whom received high dose fentanyl, the median nerve SSEP was successfully monitored. This indicates that if the changes in latency and amplitude are taken into consideration, effective monitoring can be accomplished despite high doses of fentanyl (Schubert, Peterson, Drummond, & Saidman, 1986). Infusions of sufentanil 0.5 μg/kg/hr or alfentanil 0.5 μg/kg/hr do not show a statistical change in the posterior tibial nerve SSEP (Frost, 1993).

There are other variables that occur in the operating room during surgical procedures that can affect the SEPs. These include physiologic factors, such as body temperature, systemic blood pressure, and arterial tensions of oxygen and carbon dioxide. Both hypothermia and hyperthermia can alter SEPs. Hypothermia will cause an increase in latency and a decrease in amplitude in the VEP. Hypothermia will also cause a change in morphology in the waves of the ABR (Black & Cucchiara, 1990). Hyperthermia can cause a decrease in amplitude in the SSEP (Black & Cucchiara, 1990). Irrigating fluids used in the surgical field can also cause alterations in the SEPs.

Decreases in mean systemic blood pressure to levels below cerebral autoregulation will cause progressive decreases in amplitude to a complete loss of the wave form in the SSEP (Bendo et al., 1992; Black & Cucchiara, 1990). ABR appears to be resistant to hypotension (Bendo et al., 1992; Black & Cucchiara, 1990). Sometimes during spinal surgery, changes in SSEP following the manipulation for scoliosis have been reversed with an increase in mean blood pressure, indicating that levels of hypotension considered to be safe may lead to spinal cord ischemia during the period of manipulation (Bendo et al., 1992; Black & Cucchiara, 1990).

Alterations in arterial oxygen and carbon dioxide levels will cause changes in the SEPs (Bendo et al., 1992; Black & Cucchiara, 1990). A hematocrit of 15% via hemodilution resulted in increases in latency during SSEP monitoring (Bendo et al., 1992; Black & Cucchiara, 1990).

MOTOR EVOKED POTENTIALS

Intraoperative monitoring of motor evoked potentials (MEP) is becoming more common. There are several differing techniques for monitoring intraoperative MEPs. MEPs can be recorded as an EMG following direct peripheral or cranial nerve electrical stimulation by placing recording electrodes directly in or on the innervated muscles. The electromyography (EMG) is the response of the muscle to stimulation of the motor nerve (Bendo et al., 1992). Another technique is to monitor the motor nerve tracts by using transcranial electrical motor evoked responses (tce-MER), and transcranial magnetic motor evoked responses (tcm-MER). These techniques involve transcranial electrical or magnetic stimulation and the response is measured from either peripheral nerves or muscles (Black & Cucchiara, 1990; Kalkman, Drummond, & Ribberink, 1991; Kalkman, Drummond, Kennelly et al., 1992; Kalkman, Drummond, Ribberink et al., 1992; McPherson, 1993; Nadstawek, Tanijuchi, Langenbach, & Bremer, 1992; Peterson, Drummond, & Todd, 1986).

MEPs are currently used to monitor the facial nerve during acoustic neuroma resection, microvascular decompression for hemifacial spasm, resection of cerebellopontine angle tumors, and other surgeries of the posterior fossa (Bendo, et al., 1992; Black & Cucchiara, 1990; Harner, Daube, Ebersold, & Beatty, 1987; Welna, Oliver, Daube, & Lennon, 1988). Other cranial nerves may also be monitored, including the trigeminal nerve, the spinal accessory nerve, the hypoglossal nerve, and the nerves to extraocular muscles (Black & Cucchiara, 1990). MEP monitoring can be useful in surgical procedures of the spine, such as selective dorsal rhizotomy or surgical procedures for scoliosis. Monitoring MEPs during surgeries of the spine can be used in conjunction with SSEP. SSEP monitors the sensory tracts, therefore, an injury to the motor tracts may not be demonstrated by SSEP monitoring alone. The addition of monitoring MEPs during spinal surgery may preclude the need for an intraoperative wake-up test.

MEPs are affected by drugs that interfere with the integrity of the neuromuscular junction, if the recorded response is of a muscle action potential.

The standard protocol has been that all neuromuscular blocking drugs (NMB) are avoided during surgical procedures while MEPs are being recorded. The drugs in question are the paralyzing agents used by anesthesiologist for muscle relaxation during surgical procedures. The avoidance of the use of NMB drugs may be a challenge to the anesthesiologist, especially if the anesthetic does not employ a volatile inhalation agent. Patients who are anesthetized may move in response to noxious stimuli, have involuntary muscle movement, or the patient may have movement in response to the monitoring stimulation. In the type of surgery under consideration, an inadvertent movement by the patient could be very detrimental to the outcome of the surgery. There are recent studies evaluating the use of neuromuscular blocking drugs in low doses during anesthetics while monitoring MEP. Three studies have been published recently (Adams et al., 1993; Kalkman, Drummond, Kennelly et al., 1992; McPherson, 1993; Welna et al., 1988). Two of the studies were on patients undergoing spinal surgery and one study was of a group of six patients undergoing surgery for the resection of an acoustic neuroma. In these three studies, a continuous infusion of either atracurium or vecuronium was used. The anesthesiologist adjusted the infusion's delivery rate so as to maintain two to three twitches of the train of four as monitored by the nerve stimulator. By using a continuous infusion of an intermediate acting NMB drug, the anesthesiologist can maintain close control over the degree of neuromuscular blockade and also the ability to reverse the NMB, if deemed necessary. All of the above studies indicate that under specific circumstances there was adequate monitoring of MEP. However, if one is to use intraoperative cranial nerve monitoring with extremely low levels of constant current stimulation for prognostic interpretation (Beck, Atkins, Benecke, & Brackmann, 1990), the effect of low-level muscle relaxants (neuromuscular blockade) on the EMG response and the prognostic interpretation is unknown. I strongly advise this issue be discussed between the surgeon, the anesthesiologist, and the audiologist before the surgical procedure.

When recording EMG following cranial or peripheral nerve stimulation, it appears that the anesthetic technique, except for the use of NMB, has very little influence. If the patient has preoperative abnormalities, the volatile anesthetics may influence the monitoring capabilities more than the narcotic drugs (Black & Cucchiara, 1990).

Very little data are available on the effect of anesthetic agents and monitoring intraoperative MEPs following transcranial stimulation. This type of intraoperative monitoring appears to be more sensitive to anesthetic agents than SEPs. When monitoring MEP with transcranial stimulation, whether electrical or magnetic, the general anesthetic agents may interfere with the ability to monitor motor potentials. The effects for several anesthetic agents are listed in Table 13-2. From the limited information available, it

TABLE 13-1. DRUG EFFECTS ON MEP.

Drug	Amplitude	Latency
Etomidate	No Change	↑
Fentanyl	No Change?	No Change?
Diazepam	↓	↑
Ketamine	↓	↑
Nitrous Oxide	↓	↑
Halothane	↓	↑
Isoflurane (0.5%-1.5%)	↓	↑

↑ = increase,   ↓ = decrease

Source: Adapted from "Intraoperative Neurologic Monitoring" by R. W. McPherson (p. 820) in *Principles and Practice of Anesthesiology,* M. Rogers, J. Tinker, B. Covino, and D. E. Longnecker (Eds.), 1993, St. Louis: Mosby Year Book, Inc. Copyright 1993 by Mosby Year Book, Inc. Adapted by permission.

appears that the volatile anesthetic agents will increase latency and decrease amplitude (Bendo et al., 1992; Black & Cucchiara, 1990; Calancie, Klose, Baier, & Green, 1991; Kalkman et al., 1991; McPherson 1993). At low levels of isoflurane, significant alterations in MEP occurred (Calancie et al., 1991; Kalkman et al., 1991). When isoflurane (0.2%–0.6%) was added to an already existing anesthetic there were significant alterations in tce-MER (Calancie et al., 1991; Kalkman et al., 1991). The point of interference in the neuro transmission is still under study. In a study in which the MEP was measured in the extradural space following transcranial stimulation, the addition of halothane did not significantly affect the latency or the amplitude (Laughnan et al., 1989). A significant factor in this study was that the recording electrodes were in the extradural space as opposed to muscle tissue. Nitrous oxide appears to have more of an effect on monitoring MEPs than on monitoring SEPs. Significant attenuation was found in a study done in humans using nitrous oxide (Zentner, Kiss, & Ebner, 1989). In a study with rats using 66% nitrous oxide, a significant decrease in amplitude was noted. However, at 50% nitrous oxide, a minimal change was found (Bendo et al., 1992).

Several intravenous anesthetic agents have been studied. Midazolam and propofol will cause significant decreases in amplitude with tce-MER and tcm-MER when motor responses are recorded from the tibialis anterior muscle (Kalkman, Drummond, Ribberink et al., 1992). Midazolam does not affect the latency. The interference of midazolam with transcranial stimulation is at the cortical level and not at the peripheral nerve (Schonle et al., 1989). Etomidate will cause a transient decrease in amplitude. An induction dose of thiopental has been reported to produce a loss of potentials (Bendo et al., 1992). Fentanyl has been shown to cause a decrease in amplitude (Bendo et al., 1992; Kalkman, Drummond, Ribberink et al., 1992).

Although the ability to monitor intraoperative MEPs following transcranial stimulation is very much influenced by all the anesthetic agents, it would appear that a nitrous oxide/narcotic technique allows for the most reliable recordings.

CONCLUSION

It is apparent that intraoperative monitoring is a highly valuable tool when used appropriately during surgery. Further, it is clear that anesthetic drugs can have an enormous effect on intraoperative monitoring. It is important for the audiologist, anesthesiologist, and surgeon to work together to enhance the usefulness, correctly interpret, and efficiently act on the electrophysiologic data made available by intraoperative monitoring.

REFERENCES

Adams, D. C., Emerson, R. G., Heyer, E. J., McCormick, P. C., Carmel, P. W., Stein, B. M., Farcy, J. P., & Gallo, E. J. (1993). Monitoring of intraoperative motor-evoked potentials under conditions of controlled neuromuscular blockade. *Anesthesia and Analgesia, 77*, 913–918.

Beck, D. L., Atkins, J. S., Benecke, J. E., & Brackmann, D. E. (1991). Intraoperative facial nerve monitoring: Prognostic aspects during acoustic tumor removal. *Otolaryngology—Head and Neck Surgery, 104*, 780–782.

Bendo, A., Kass, I., Hartung, J., & Cottrell, J. (1992). Neurophysiology and neuroanesthesia. In P. Barash, B. Cullen, & R. Stoelting (Eds.), *Clinical anesthesia* (pp. 871–918). Philadelphia: J. B. Lippincott Company.

Black, S., & Cucchiara, R. (1990). Neurologic monitoring. In R. Miller (Ed.), *Anesthesia* (pp. 1185–1207). New York: Churchill Livingstone.

Calancie, B., Klose, K. J., Baier, S., & Green, B. A. (1991). Isoflurane-induced attenuation of motor evoked potentials caused by electrical motor cortex stimulation during surgery. *Journal of Neurosurgery, 74*, 879–904.

Frost, E. (1993). Electroencephalography and evoked potential monitoring. In L. Saidman & N. Smith (Eds.), *Monitoring in anesthesia* (pp. 203–223). Boston: Butterworth-Heinemann.

Grundy, B. L. (1980). Fentanyl alters somatosensory cortical evoked potentials. (Abstract). *Anesthesia & Analgesia, 59*, 544.

Grundy, B. L. (1983). Intraoperative monitoring of sensory-evoked potentials. *Anesthesiology, 58,* 72–87.

Grundy, B. L., Jannetta, P. J., Procopia, P. T., Lina, A., Boston, J. R., & Doyle, E. (1982). Intraoperative monitoring of brain-stem auditory evoked potentials. *Journal of Neurosurgery, 57,* 674–681.

Harner, S. G., Daube, J. R., Ebersold, M. J., & Beatty, C. W. (1987). Improved preservation of facial nerve function with use of electrical monitoring during removal of acoustic neuromas. *Mayo Clinic Proceedings, 62,* 92–102.

Hogan, K. (1992). Neuroanesthetic techniques for intraoperative monitoring. In J. Kartush & K. Bouchard (Eds.), *Neuromonitoring in otology and head and neck surgery* (pp. 61–77). New York: Raven Press Ltd.

Kalkman, C. J., Drummond, J. C., Kennelly, N. A., Patel, P. M., & Partridge, B. L. (1992). Intraoperative monitoring of tibialis anterior muscle motor evoked responses to transcranial electrical stimulation during partial neuromuscular blockade. *Anesthesia & Analgesia, 75,* 584–589.

Kalkman, C. J., Drummond, J. C., & Ribberink, A. A. (1991). Low concentrations of isoflurane abolish motor evoked responses to transcranial electrical stimulation during nitrous oxide/opioid anesthesia in humans. *Anesthesia & Analgesia, 73,* 410–415.

Kalkman, C. J., Drummond, J. C., Ribberink, A. A., Patel, P. M., Sano, T., & Bickford, R. G. (1992). Effects of propofol, etomidate, midazalam, and fentanyl on motor evoked reponses to transcranial electrical or magnetic stimulation in humans. *Anesthesiology, 76,* 502–509.

Laughnan, B. A., Anderson, S. K., Hetreed, M. A., Weston, P. F., Boyd, S. G., & Hall, G. M. (1989). Effects of halothane on motor evoked potential recorded in the extradural space. (Abstract). *British Journal of Anaesthesia, 63,* 561–564.

McPherson, R. W. (1993). Intraoperative neurologic monitoring. In M. Rogers, J. Tinker, B. Covino, & D. E. Longnecker (Eds.), *Principles and practice of anesthesiology* (pp. 803–821). St. Louis: Mosby-Year Book, Inc.

Nadstawek, J., Tanijuchi, M., Langenbach, U., & Bremer, F. (1992). Effects of four intravenous anesthetic agents on motor evoked potentials elicited by magnetic transcranial stimulation. (Abstract). *Anesthesiology, 77,* A500.

Navartnarajah, M., Thorton, C., Heneghan, C. P. H., Bateman, E., & Jones, J. G. (1983). Effect of etomidate on the auditory evoked response in man. *Proceedings of the Anesthetic Research Society, 55,* 1157P.

Pathak, K. S., Brown, R. H., Cascorbi, H. F., & Nash, C. L. (1984). Effects of fentanyl and morphine on intraoperative somatosensory cortical-evoked potentials. *Anesthesia & Analgesia, 63,* 833–837.

Peterson, D. O., Drummond, J. C., & Todd, M. M. (1986). Effects of halothane, enflurane, isoflurane and nitrous oxide on somatosensory evoked potentials in humans. *Anesthesiology, 65,* 35–40.

Schonle, P. W., Isenberg, C., Crozier, T. A., Dressler, D., Machetanz, T., & Conrad, B. (1989). Changes in transcranially evoked motor reponses in man by midazalam, a short acting benzodiazepine. *Neuroscience Letters, 101,* 321–324.

Schubert, A., Peterson, D. O., Drummond, J. C., & Saidman, L. J. (1986). The effect of high dose fentanyl on human median nerve somatosensory evoked responses. (Abstract). *Anesthesia & Analgesia, 65,* S1–S170.

Stoelting, R. K., & Miller, R. (Eds.). (1984). *Basics of anesthesia*. New York: Churchill Livingstone.

Welna, J. O., Oliver, S. B., Daube, J. R., & Lennon, R. L. (1988). Effect of partial neuromuscular blockade on intraoperative electromyography in patients undergoing resection of acoustic neuroma. (Abstract). *Anesthesiology, 69,* A636.

Zentner, J., Kiss, I., & Ebner, A. (1989). Influence of anesthetics—nitrous oxide in particular—on electromyographic response evoked by transcranial electrical stimulation of the cortex. *Neurosurgery, 24,* 253–256.

■ INDEX ■